AMERICAN ACADEMY OF PEDIATRICS

Managing Infectious Diseases in Child Care and Schools

A Quick Reference Guide

Editors

Susan S. Aronson, MD, FAAP

Timothy R. Shope, MD, MPH, FAAP

AAP Department of Marketing and Publications Staff

Maureen DeRosa, MPA
Director, Department of Marketing and Publications

Mark Grimes
Director, Division of Product Development

Jeff Mahony
Manager, Product Development

Sandi King
Director, Division of Publishing and Production Services

Kate Larson
Manager, Editorial Services

Jason Crase
Editorial Specialist

Leesa Levin-Doroba
Manager, Print Production Services

Linda Diamond
Manager, Graphic Design

Peggy Mulcahy
Graphic Designer

Jill Ferguson
Director, Division of Marketing and Sales

Susan Thompson
Manager, Consumer Product Marketing and Sales

Library of Congress Control Number: 2004101464

ISBN: 1-58110-134-1

MA0278

The recommendations in this publication do not indicate an exclusive course of treatment or serve as a standard of medical care. Variations, taking into account individual circumstances, may be appropriate. The views expressed in this publication are those of the authors and do not reflect the official policy or position of the Department of the Navy, Department of Defense, or the United States Government.

Reviewers/Contributors

Editors
Susan S. Aronson, MD, FAAP
Timothy R. Shope, MD, MPH, FAAP

AAP Board of Directors Reviewer
Edgar O. Ledbetter, MD, FAAP

Technical Reviewers
Danette S. Glassy, MD, FAAP
Dennis L. Murray, MD, FAAP
Judith T. Romano, MD, FAAP
Howard L. Taras, MD, FAAP

American Academy of Pediatrics
Errol R. Alden, MD, FAAP
Executive Director/CEO

Joe M. Sanders, Jr, MD, FAAP
Immediate Past Executive Director

Roger F. Suchyta, MD, FAAP
Associate Executive Director

Maureen DeRosa, MPA
Director, Department of Marketing and Publications

Mark Grimes
Director, Division of Product Development

Jeff Mahony
Manager, Product Development

Thomas F. Tonniges, MD, FAAP
Director, Department of Community Pediatrics

Sunnah Kim, MS, RN
Director, Division of Community Health Services

Laura Aird, MS
Manager, Child Care Initiatives

Michael San Filippo
Publications Specialist

Lauren Kotch
Sheryl Nelson, MS
Healthy Child Care America Staff

Writer
Jane Cotler, MS, RN

Table of Contents

Foreword

In the United States, more than two-thirds of children younger than 6 years, and almost all children older than 6 years, spend significant time in child care and school settings outside of the home. Exposure to groups of children increases the risk of infectious diseases. This fact has important personal, public health, economic, and social consequences. The intent of this book is to provide an easy-to-use reference for those who are responsible for the prevention and management of infectious diseases in child care and school settings—caregivers/teachers, pediatric health professionals, and parents.

Caregivers/teachers will find this book offers easy-to-read explanations for how infectious diseases spread, how to prepare for inevitable illness, and how to incorporate measures that limit any excess burden of illness associated with group activities. The Signs and Symptoms Chart (Chapter 6) will help nonmedical professionals know what certain symptoms might mean. The set of fact sheets (Chapter 7, "Quick Reference Sheets") describes specific types of infectious diseases in common terms, with guidance about how they spread and what needs to be done by caregivers/teachers, children, and families when someone in the group has a disease. By using this book as a handy reference, caregivers/teachers can feel more confident and act more appropriately in making decisions about inclusion and exclusion of ill children and in seeking advice from medical professionals when necessary to reduce the burden of infectious diseases to other children and staff.

Pediatricians and other health professionals will find this book helpful as a reference that facilitates communication with caregivers/teachers. Pediatric health professionals are the primary source of information for caregivers/teachers about the management of infectious diseases for individual children and the implications of these infections for groups of children and the adults who care for them. Pediatric health professionals can use the content of the book to identify exclusion and inclusion recommendations, supplement their communications with educators about infectious diseases of patients, and augment their instructions for the care of the child for parents and caregivers/teachers involved in the child's care. They can also use the content of the book to identify the need for linking caregivers/teachers with public health authorities when needed.

Parents will benefit from the content of this book because it will provide a common means for communication between pediatric health professionals and caregivers/teachers that is based on the best available medical information. Additionally, parents will benefit from the quick reference sheets, which may be copied and sent home. These sheets can be used to describe a condition or infection affecting their child or the group of children to which their child is exposed.

This book also addresses the controversial subject of exclusion and return-to-care criteria. Controversy exists because caregivers/teachers, pediatric health professionals, and parents frequently disagree about which conditions require exclusion. For example, children with runny noses may be unnecessarily excluded but others with diarrhea may be allowed to stay, when they in fact may pose a greater infection risk. Adding to the confusion, each state health department and licensing agency has unique rules or exclusion criteria for determining which symptoms, diseases, and conditions require exclusion from child care or school.

The recommendations in this book are based on the best available medical information as determined by the American Academy of Pediatrics. The exclusion criteria in this book are generally much more detailed than existing guidelines and can be followed without conflict with existing rules or regulations. It is our hope that policy makers incorporate the exclusion and return-to-care recommendations in this book as they move toward revising their state policies and regulations.

—Susan S. Aronson, MD, FAAP
Timothy R. Shope, MD, MPH, FAAP

About This Book

Managing Infectious Diseases in Child Care and Schools: A Quick Reference Guide is a tool to encourage common understanding among caregivers/teachers, families, and health professionals about infectious diseases in group care settings for children. This easy reference guide identifies

- The role of caregivers/teachers, families, and health professionals in preventing and controlling the spread of communicable infections
- Symptoms of infections commonly found in group settings for children
- How infections are spread (routes of transmission)
- When to seek medical attention
- Inclusion and exclusion criteria
- Sample forms for communications involving caregivers/teachers, parents/guardians, and health professionals

Others who are involved with group care settings for children, such as state licensing professionals and policy makers, will find this guide helpful when writing and implementing regulations, updating state policies, and educating others about these issues.

The information in this quick reference guide is based on the latest recommendations addressing health and safety in group care settings from the following organizations:
- American Academy of Pediatrics
- American Public Health Association
- US Department of Health and Human Services
- Centers for Disease Control and Prevention

For a general guide on caring for young children, refer to

American Academy of Pediatrics. *Caring for Your Baby and Young Child: Birth to Age 5.* Shelov SP, Hannemann RE, eds. 4th ed. New York, NY: Bantam Books; 2004

The references for the content of the quick reference guide are

American Academy of Pediatrics, American Public Health Association, National Resource Center for Health and Safety in Child Care. *Caring for Our Children: National Health and Safety Performance Standards: Guidelines for Out-of-Home Child Care Programs.* 2nd ed. Elk Grove Village, IL: American Academy of Pediatrics; 2002. Available at: http://nrc.uchsc.edu/CFOC/index.html. Accessed June 10, 2004

American Academy of Pediatrics. *Red Book: 2003 Report of the Committee on Infectious Diseases.* Pickering LK, ed. 26th ed. Elk Grove Village, IL: American Academy of Pediatrics; 2003

CHAPTER 1

Introduction:
Keeping Children Healthy

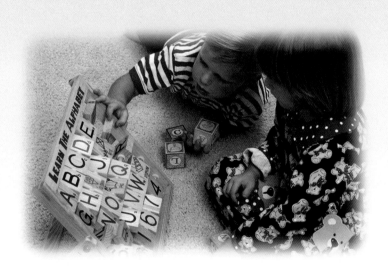

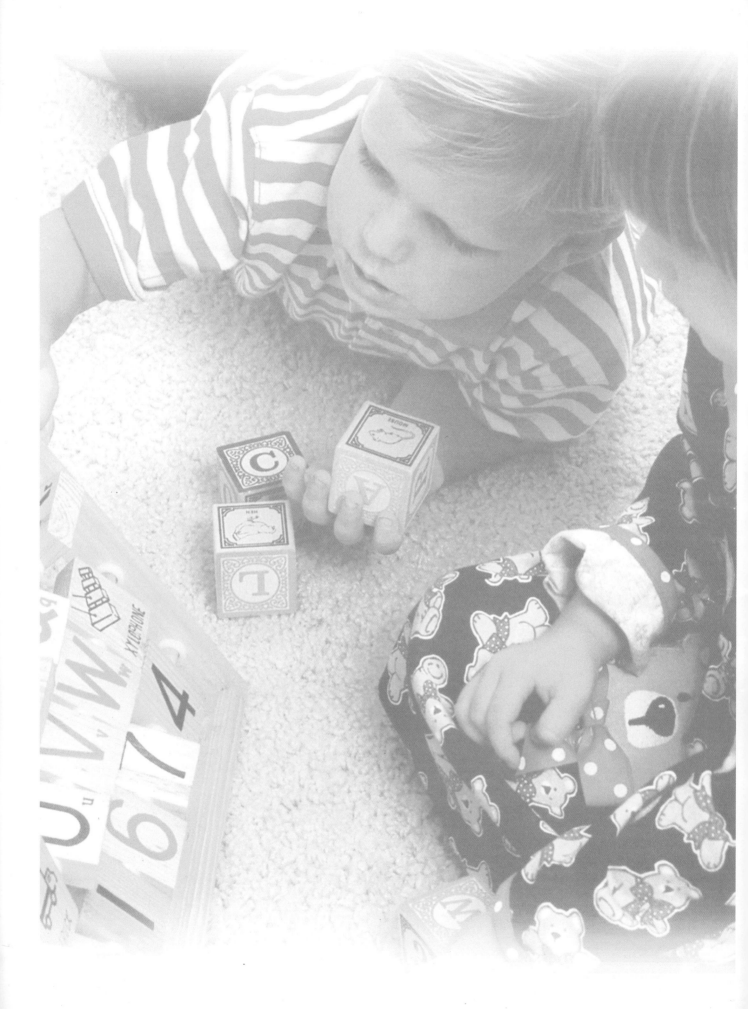

Introduction: Keeping Children Healthy

Keeping children healthy is a goal of caregivers/teachers, families, and health professionals. However, there are many factors that can make staying healthy a challenge. When children first enter group settings, their immune systems are still developing and they have not yet been exposed to many common germs that cause infection (eg, viruses, bacteria, parasites, fungi). Infants and toddlers have high hand-to-mouth activity. They play and eat close together, so they easily pass germs to each other. In general, sending home *(excluding)* mildly ill children is not an effective way to control the spread of most germs. Many infections are spread by individuals who are not ill (ie, before or after an illness) or never become ill. (Some ill children need to be excluded for reasons apart from reducing the spread of illness. See Chapter 5, "Recognizing the Ill Child: Inclusion/Exclusion Criteria," on page 25.) All of these factors make infections in group care environments common and fast spreading.

A child with a contagious or communicable illness has an infection that can be passed to another person. However, common respiratory infections most often cause coughs and colds that are relatively harmless and resolve without treatment. These infections are less frequent when a child grows older and as the child spends more time in group settings. These common infections stimulate the immune system to protect the child as the child grows up. Nevertheless, common, minor illnesses can cause some short-term discomfort for the child and lost work for the family member who stays home to care for the ill child. Therefore, the frequency and severity of these common infections should be reduced as much as possible.

A small number of infections among children in group care settings can cause serious disease. Some have a high potential for rapid spread. These illnesses are covered in Chapter 5, "Recognizing the Ill Child: Inclusion/Exclusion Criteria," on page 25. Following proper infection control procedures (see Chapter 3, "Infection Control Measures," on page 11) will reduce the spread of mild respiratory infections as well as infections that may be more serious.

Germs and infections can spread by
- Coughing or sneezing, which sends infectious droplets from a person who has the disease into the air that susceptible children and adults then breathe into their bodies
- Touching infectious body fluids or secretions (eg, mucus, saliva, blood, urine, stool) of someone who has germs that cause disease
- Touching an object previously contaminated by someone with germs from infectious body fluids or secretions

It is important for families, caregivers/teachers, and health professionals to work together to promote healthy behaviors and prevent infections and diseases.

Parents/guardians can
- Seek pediatric care that is accessible, continuous, comprehensive, coordinated, compassionate, culturally competent, and family centered. Such a source of health care is known as a *medical home* (see www.medicalhomeinfo.org). When this is not achievable, families should seek care from a source that most closely meets the medical home concept in their community. A medical home is provided by a group of pediatric physicians (pediatricians or family practice physicians) who provide collaborative care with nurse practitioners, or by pediatric professionals in a private setting or health department clinic.
- Choose to breastfeed babies. Research shows that breast milk, with its unique mixture of fatty acids, lactose, amino acids, vitamins, minerals, enzymes, and other components, helps protect infants from illness.
- Make sure their children receive recommended immunizations and checkups from a source of pediatric health care.
  ~ Most recommended vaccines are required for attendance in child care programs and schools. The risk of exposure to vaccine-preventable diseases is increased when children gather in groups for any reason.
  ~ Unless medical exemptions or contraindications exist or children have received religious or philosophical exemptions, immunization records should demonstrate that the child received the vaccines shown in the current *Recommended Childhood and Adolescent Immunization Schedule,* which is published on an annual basis, typically in January (available online at www.cispimmunize.org and www.aapredbook.org).
  ~ Children who have not received recommended age-appropriate immunizations before enrollment should be immunized as soon as possible, and the series should be completed according to the catch-up immunization schedules for children and adolescents who start late or who are more than 1 month behind (available online at www.cispimmunize.org and www.aapredbook.org).
- Communicate with the staff in the children's group care setting about possible illness in their children.
- Plan to pick up children promptly and care for them in a comfortable place away from others when children are too ill to remain in the group care setting.

- Talk with the children's health professionals about diagnosis and care when children are moderately or severely ill or possibly have an illness that poses a risk to others in the group care setting.

Caregivers/teachers can
- Review each child's health record with the parent/guardian at time of enrollment, clarifying questions about the child's health with the parent/guardian and the child's health professional.
- Support mothers who choose to breastfeed their babies. Research shows that breast milk, with its unique mixture of fatty acids, lactose, amino acids, vitamins, minerals, enzymes, and other components, helps protect infants from illness.
- Enforce the policy that children must have up-to-date immunizations for participation in the program; exceptions (eg, medical, religious, or philosophical exemptions) should be properly documented as required by state law. If a child does not receive immunizations due to the family's beliefs, the program should notify the parents/guardians about the risk of spread of preventable diseases. In such situations, the program should require that the parents sign a waiver of the program's responsibility for exposure of the child to increased risk from infectious diseases. Also, the program should be prepared to exclude unimmunized children from the facility if a vaccine-preventable disease occurs in the facility to which their lack of vaccination makes them more susceptible.
- Work with families and appropriate professionals to develop plans to care for children with special needs and other children who are unable to participate in the regular program.
- Pay special attention to children who have increased risk from infectious disease—those who are incompletely immunized or unimmunized, do not have a medical home and use emergency departments resulting in fragmented or sporadic medical care, or travel outside the United States. Also, consider at increased risk children who have family members who travel outside the United States, who are or have been in prison, or who are drug users.
- Provide accessible sinks with warm water, soap, disposable towels, hand lotion, and easy-to-understand posted instructions to facilitate good hand washing and hygiene practices for each group of children within the area where activities take place.
- Model good hand washing and hygiene practices and encourage children to do the same.
- Help families develop a care plan to use when their children are ill.
- Notify families when children become ill. The health department should also be notified if children possibly have a contagious disease that might pose a risk for others in a group care setting. Such notification might be coordinated with the child's health professional. However, caregivers/teachers must recognize their special duty to report an outbreak or that a serious illness has been diagnosed in a child who is enrolled in the group care setting. Often, the physician's report of the diagnosis of the disease does not include consideration of the exposure of others who are not members of the child's family.
- Make sure staff are healthy by keeping their immunizations and other recommended preventive care services up to date.
- Work on communicating effectively with families and health professionals. Try to understand how difficult it is for families to deal with illnesses in their children while attending to their other adult responsibilities. Also, try to understand how the usually fast-paced work of pediatric health care may lead to misunderstandings. What usually works best is to provide a clear, brief statement of what you have observed without telling the health professional what tests or treatments you think are necessary. Use a written note that the parent can take to the health professional to inform about your observations, and ask for a return note when the situation seems unclear to you. Avoid asking for routine notes for return after illnesses when the child seems well. When there is a communication problem that involves a health professional, caregivers/teachers should ask the office staff of the health professional about the best way to communicate to get help from the health professional. Sometimes effective communication requires a direct contact between the caregiver/teacher and the health professional. When an individual child is involved, such direct contact always requires written parental consent.

Health professionals can
- Support mothers who choose to breastfeed their babies, and endorse breastfeeding as an important preventive health care strategy. Research shows that breast milk, with its unique mixture of fatty acids, lactose, amino acids, vitamins, minerals, enzymes, and other components, helps protect infants from illness.
- Keep good immunization records and implement reminder/recall systems to ensure each child is age-appropriately immunized and up to date with all preventive care services.
- Provide management instructions for ill children not only to families but also to other caregivers/teachers who are responsible for giving treatment to the child at any time during the day. Caregivers/teachers should not be expected to rely on relayed communications from families that can be misunderstood.
- Help to develop a plan for care of children with special needs related to chronic or acute infections and for at-risk children with exemptions from immunizations.
- Provide educational sessions on health topics for families and caregivers/teachers.

- Educate families and caregivers/teachers about appropriate inclusion and exclusion practices.
- Help determine the severity of children's illnesses and what levels of illness each child care program and school can manage with available personnel and other resources.
- Sensitively respond to questions asked by families and caregivers/teachers about the implications of infectious diseases for children's participation in a group care setting. Avoid suggesting that the child's participation in a group care setting is necessarily the source of a particular infectious illness. Community exposure and family exposure, as well as exposure in a group care setting, are all potential sources of any individual illness. Be cautious about making negative comments to families about the care provided by the caregivers/teachers who are responsible not only for a particular child, but for the entire group of children.

- Provide thoughtful advice for the family of a child with recurrent infections. Assess whether the child is actually having more frequent or more severe infectious diseases than is typical for the age of the child. If so, consider asking for parental consent for discussing preventive measures with the caregivers/teachers, such as more frequent and more careful hand washing for children and staff, better hygiene in the diapering and toileting areas, and better ventilation of rooms. Inquire about whether the facility has access to a health consultant who might assess the situation at the group care setting to see whether any additional measures would be helpful.

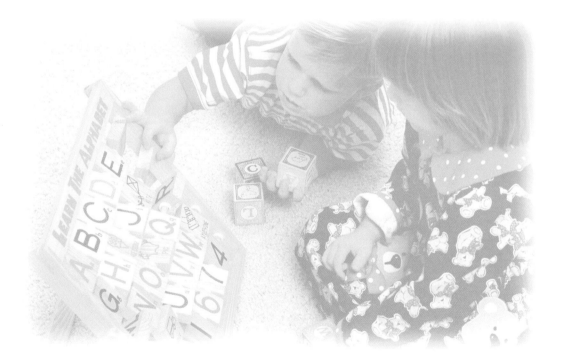

CHAPTER 2

Infection Overview

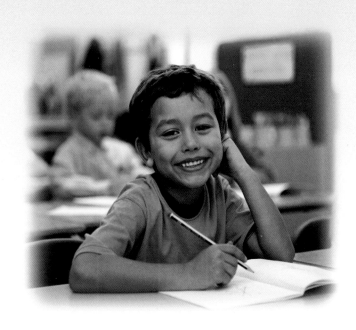

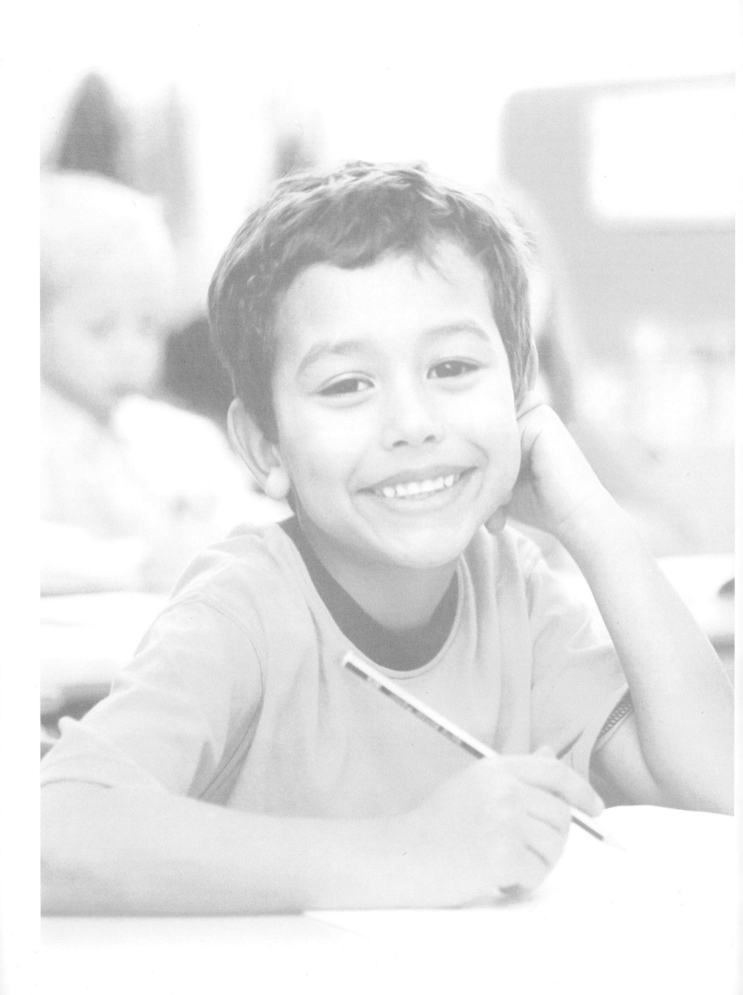

Infection Overview

In group care settings, close personal contact and inadequate hygiene of young children provide good opportunities for the spread (transmission) of germs. *Germ* is the common term for a large variety of microbial agents that can grow in or on people. Some are harmless or even helpful. *Infection* is the term usually used to describe a situation in which a germ causes disease. Germs include bacteria, viruses, parasites, and fungi. Although not technically correct, sometimes infection is used to describe invasion of the body by higher organisms called *parasites* (eg, worms, insects).

Infection Spread by Direct Contact With People or Objects

Infection can spread through direct contact with an infected area of someone's body or contact with contaminated hands or any substance or surface that holds infectious material (eg, mucus, diaper changing table). Many objects can absorb, retain, and transport germs. In child care and school settings, the surfaces of floors, activity and food tables, diaper changing tables, doorknobs, toilet room surfaces, toys, and fabric objects may have a lot of germs on them if they are not properly cleaned and sanitized. Direct head-to-head touching, shared hats and hairbrushes, or storing jackets so they touch each other can spread infestations such as lice. Skin-to-skin or skin-to-bedding touching can spread impetigo and scabies. Mouth-to-mouth kissing can spread respiratory germs of all types.

Infection Spread by the Fecal-Oral Route

Children in diapers at any age constitute a high risk for the spread of gastrointestinal infections through contamination by microscopic amounts of the material produced by a bowel movement. The medical term for this substance is *fecal matter* or *stool*. With typical frequent diaper changing and mouthing behaviors, hands, floors, toilet and faucet handles, diaper changing areas, toys, and countertops frequently are contaminated with fecal matter. Germs can spread by the fecal-oral route if the infected person does not perform hand washing after toileting or before food preparation or if anyone eats food contaminated with disease-causing germs.

Infection Spread by the Respiratory Route

Airborne droplets that have germs from the respiratory tract can spread by breathing the air close to someone who has coughed or sneezed or touching surfaces that have moist secretions from an infected person's nose, eye, mouth, or throat. The most common surfaces that spread airborne droplets are hands. Teaching children to cover their mouths or noses with their hands when they cough or sneeze actually *helps* to spread germs. Hands touch everywhere all the time. Unless good hand washing is performed right after using hands to cover a sneeze or cough, the hands will spread germs.

It is best to use a disposable paper nasal tissue to cover a cough or sneeze, and then perform good hand washing before touching anything else. This is not always possible. Few people can get a disposable paper nasal tissue to the right place quickly enough to do the job. Teach children that it is better to direct a sudden cough or sneeze to an empty space on the floor (where children are not crawling) or use an elbow or a shoulder as a barrier (ie, "giving a sneeze or cough a cold shoulder"). Wherever the cough or sneeze was directed becomes contaminated, of course. Do not cuddle an infant on the shoulder used to catch a cough or sneeze without a clean covering in that location. Children with respiratory infections tend to contaminate their hands, forearms, shirtsleeves, and other objects with mucus from their noses, eyes, and throats. All of these surfaces play a role in the spread of infection.

Infection Spread Through Blood, Urine, and Saliva

Contact with blood and other body fluids of another person requires more intimate exposure than usually occurs in group settings. Some infections are spread through contact of contaminated blood with the mucous membrane or a cut that lets the germs into the body. While theoretically possible, infected children are unlikely to spread infection by biting in a group setting. To spread an infection in this way requires blood in the mouth (ie, drawing blood from the victim or transferring blood to the victim from the biter's bleeding gums). Many child bites do not break the skin. When a bite does break the skin, the mouth of the biter does not usually stay on the victim long enough for blood to transfer. Few children have bleeding gums. Routine infant and child immunization against a virus that can spread through saliva (ie, hepatitis B virus) has virtually eliminated the risk of transmission of this disease through biting.

Following standard precautions to remove blood from the environment safely prevents transmission of blood-borne germs. Because it is impossible to know who might have a blood-borne disease, routine use of standard precautions protects everyone against the spread of human immunodeficiency virus, hepatitis B, hepatitis C, and hepatitis D.

Saliva and urine often contain viruses long after a child has recovered from an illness. Good hand washing and standard precautions will help prevent the spread of these viruses.

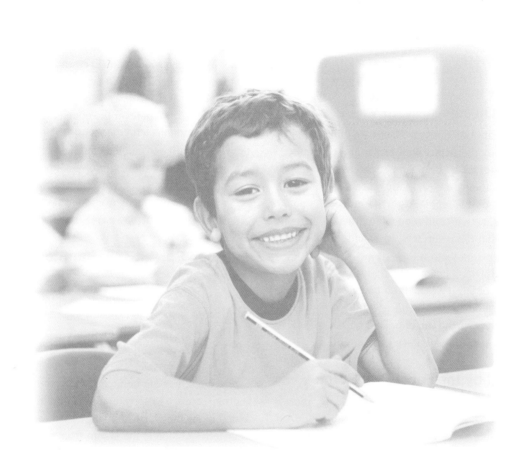

CHAPTER 3

Infection Control
Measures

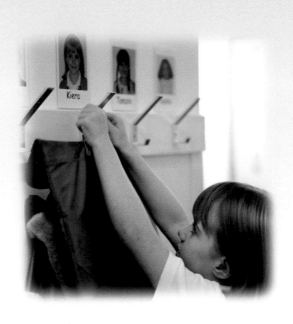

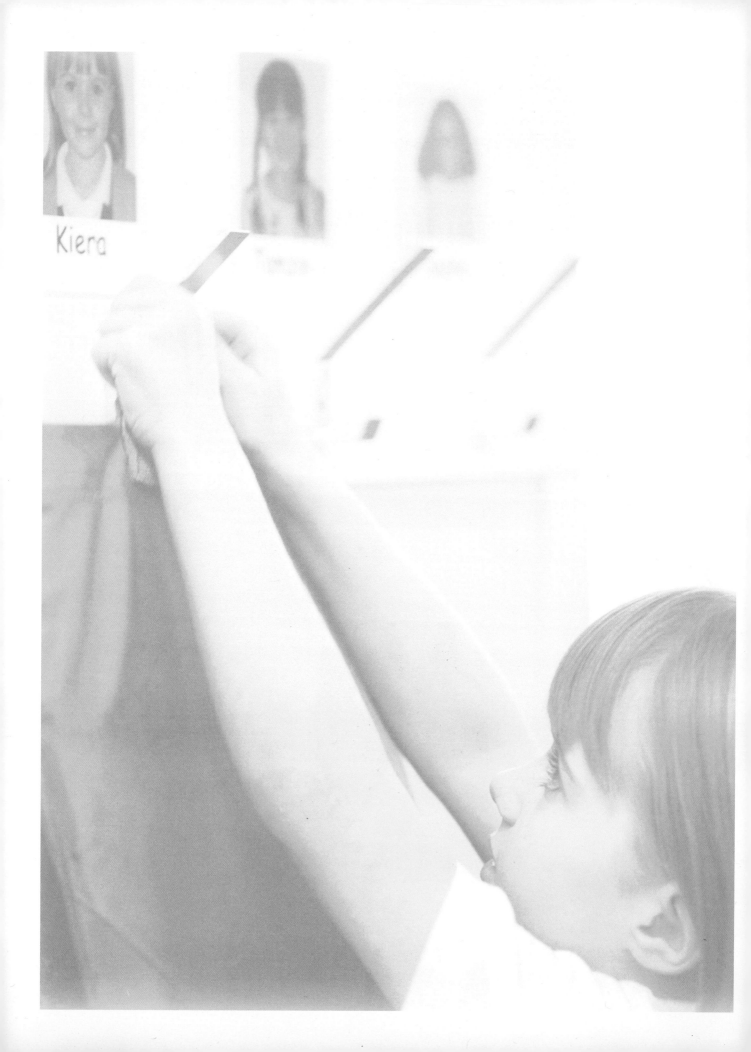

Kiera

Infection Control Measures

Administration and Consultation

Caregivers/teachers in all group settings (home-based family child care, centers, and schools) should set up an environment to promote healthful practices and periodically obtain expert advice on corrections that are likely to prevent disease. Written policies are an essential element of infection control.

Setting Up a Healthful Environment for Children

All facilities should have written policies and procedures that define and ensure a hygienic environment in the following manner:

- Hand washing
  - ~ Sinks located in each area where activities take place
  - ~ Each sink provided with warm running water, liquid soap, disposable towels, hand lotion, and whatever else is needed to facilitate frequent hand washing (eg, safe stools for smaller children)
  - ~ Monitoring of hand washing for all adults and children at the times and by the methods listed on pages 17 and 18
- Toilet areas
  - ~ Sanitary.
  - ~ Equipped with child-sized toilets or access to steps and modified toilet seats.
  - ~ Children who need assistance with toileting should not be allowed in toilet or bathroom facilities without direct visual supervision.
- Diaper changing areas
  - ~ Sanitary
  - ~ Located away from food preparation areas and near hand washing sinks
  - ~ Contain posted diaper changing procedures
  - ~ Contain surfaces that are nonporous and sanitized between uses
- Routine environmental sanitation (See chart on page 14 for frequency for all surfaces.)
  - ~ Adhere to appropriate hand and personal hygiene for children and staff (see "Hand Washing Steps" on page 17).
  - ~ Clean/sanitize all toys.
  - ~ Clean/sanitize tables, including those used for play and for eating.
  - ~ Clean/disinfect spills of blood or body fluids.
  - ~ Disinfect floors.
  - ~ Cover sandboxes.
  - ~ Ensure pets are appropriately enclosed and their enclosures kept clean of waste.
  - ~ Ensure staff wash hands before and after handling any animal, and after handling animal waste.
  - ~ Provide separate and sanitary sleep equipment for each child.
- Food preparation
  - ~ Food should be handled in a safe and appropriate way to prevent bacterial growth and contamination.
  - ~ Staff who have symptoms of illness (eg, vomiting, diarrhea, infectious skin lesions that cannot be covered, nasal discharge that requires wiping while doing food-related activities) should not be responsible for food preparation.
  - ~ Staff whose primary function is the preparation of food should not change diapers.
  - ~ Except in home-based care, staff who work with diapered children should not prepare or serve food for older groups of children.
  - ~ When staff who are caring for infants and toddlers are responsible for changing diapers, they should handle food only for the infants and toddlers in their groups and only after thoroughly washing their hands.

Health Consultant

All programs in which children routinely spend time should have a health consultant to

- Assist in the development and implementation of written policies for prevention and control of communicable diseases.
- Do site visits to spot and help correct hazards and risky practices and provide health education to children, child care providers, and families. Facilities with infants should seek services from a health consultant at least monthly, and all others at least quarterly. See Chapter 8, "Role of the Health Consultant in Child Care and Schools," on page 131 for more information.

Written Policies

All child care facilities and schools should have written policies that describe

- Environmental hygiene
- Inclusion and exclusion for children and staff illnesses
- Families' responsibility to share information about illnesses in children
- The need to notify local health authorities of certain communicable diseases involving children or staff
- Accurate record keeping and tracking for immunizations and other routine preventive health care services
- The need to identify the child's source of routine, comprehensive health care, known as the medical home

Cleaning and Sanitizing Chart

Area	Clean	Sanitize	Frequency
Classroom/Child Care/Food Areas			
Countertops/tabletops, floors, doorknobs, and cabinet handles	X	X	Daily and when soiled
Food preparation/service surfaces	X	X	Before/after contact with food activity; between preparation of raw and cooked foods
Carpets and large area rugs	X		Vacuum daily when children are not present. Clean with a carpet-cleaning method approved by the local health authority. Clean carpets only when children will not be present until carpet is dry. Clean carpets at least monthly in infant areas, at least every 3 months in other areas, and when soiled.
Small rugs	X		Shake outdoors or vacuum daily. Launder weekly.
Utensils, surfaces/toys that go in the mouth or have been in contact with saliva or other body fluids	X	X	After each child's use or use disposable, one-time utensils or toys.
Toys that are not contaminated with body fluids. Dress-up clothes not worn on the head. Sheets/pillowcases, individual cloth towels (if used), combs/hairbrushes, washcloths, and machine-washable cloth toys. (None of these items should be shared among children.)	X		Weekly and when visibly soiled
Blankets, sleeping bags, cubbies	X		Monthly and when soiled
Hats	X		After each child's use or use disposable hats that only one child wears
Cribs and crib mattresses	X		Weekly, before use by different child, and whenever soiled or wet
Phone receivers	X	X	Weekly
Toilet and Diapering Areas			
Hand washing sinks, faucets, surrounding counters, soap dispensers, doorknobs	X	X	Daily and when soiled
Toilet seats, toilet handles, doorknobs or cubicle handles, floors	X	X	Daily or immediately if visibly soiled
Toilet bowls	X	X	Daily
Changing tables, potty chairs (Use of potty chairs in child care is discouraged because of high risk of contamination.)	X	X	After each child's use
General Facility			
Mops and cleaning rags	X	X	Before and after a day of use, wash mops/rags in detergent and water, rinse in water, immerse in sanitizing solution, and wring as dry as possible. After cleaning and sanitizing, hang mops and rags to dry.
Waste and diaper containers	X		Daily
Any surface contaminated with body fluids (eg, saliva, mucus, vomit, urine, stool, blood)	X	X	Immediately using standard precautions as specified in *Caring for Our Children*, Standard 3.026

Adapted from National Association for the Education of Young Children. *Keeping Healthy.* 1999, as found in American Academy of Pediatrics, American Public Health Association, National Resource Center for Health and Safety in Child Care. *Caring for Our Children: National Health and Safety Performance Standards: Guidelines for Out-of-Home Child Care Programs.* 2nd ed. Elk Grove Village, IL: American Academy of Pediatrics; 2002:106. Available at: http://nrc.uchsc.edu/CFOC/index.html. Accessed June 10, 2004

Sanitation, Disinfection, and Maintenance

Routine Cleaning, Sanitizing, and Disinfecting of Contaminated Surfaces

These techniques can help reduce the spread of germs in child care and school environments. The definitions of these terms and techniques for their use follow:

- **Routine cleaning:** using detergents or abrasive cleaners and rinsing with water to remove surface soil.
- **Sanitizing:** removing filth or soil and small amounts of certain germs. For a surface to be considered sanitary, the surface must be cleaned first and then an additional sanitizer solution must be applied to reduce the number of germs to such a level that disease transmission by that surface is unlikely. This procedure is less rigorous than disinfecting and is applicable to a wide variety of routine housekeeping procedures.
  - ~ Many different types of sanitizing solutions are available.
  - ~ Follow the instructions on the manufacturer's label for correct use.
  - ~ Products that are registered with the US Environmental Protection Agency (EPA) as *detergent-disinfectant* or *hospital-grade* germicides may be used for sanitizing.
  - ~ Avoid products that are labeled as toxic for children.
  - ~ Be cautious of industrial products advertised as "having germicidal action" or "killing germs." They may not have the same effectiveness as bleach and water or EPA-approved hospital-grade germicides.
  - ~ Consult with your local health department or regulatory licensing authority for any product other than bleach.
    - ❖ Surface sanitizing method.
      - ◦ Household bleach is inexpensive, relatively safe, and easy to use and can be mixed as follows:
        - – Mix ¼ cup of household bleach to 1 gallon of tap water (or 1 tablespoon of household bleach to 1 quart of water) for a 1:64 dilution. Because chlorine evaporates from bleach and is weakened by sunlight and heat, this minimal dilution may become too diluted to be effective if not made fresh daily from the stock bottle of household bleach. Freshly purchased stock supplies should be used within a few months so they, too, do not become too weak to be effective when diluted.
        - – To sanitize with the freshly made 1:64 dilution of bleach, spray the diluted solution on the surface until glossy. Leave the bleach solution on the surface for at least 2 minutes before wiping it off with a clean paper towel, or allow it to air-dry.

- ❖ Dipping methods for sanitizing dishes and toys also are useful.
  - ◦ Follow the manufacturer's instructions on the containers for products other than bleach for this method.
  - ◦ Household bleach
    - – Mix 1.5 teaspoons of household bleach per gallon of water (100 parts per million chlorine) that is not less than 75°F.
    - – Immerse the object to be sanitized for at least 2 minutes.
    - – Allow the object to air-dry.
  - ◦ Hot water immersion
    - – Completely immerse in hot water at 170°F for not less than 30 seconds.
    - – Air-dry.
- **Disinfecting:** eliminating virtually all germs from surfaces through the use of chemicals registered with the US EPA as *disinfectants* or physical agents (eg, heat).

Prevention of Disease Transmission

Baseline routine frequency of cleaning and sanitation can be found in the chart on page 14. Frequency of cleaning and sanitation should be increased when there are

- Outbreaks of illness
- Known contamination
- Visible soil, blood, or other body fluids
- Recommendations by the health department to control certain infectious diseases

Fecal bacteria in the environment have been shown to increase during outbreaks of diarrheal illnesses. Health officials may recommend a more frequent cleaning schedule in certain areas, depending on the nature of the problem.

Common Sanitation Issues

Environmental Surfaces and Equipment

Because children will touch any reachable surface (including floors), all surfaces may be contaminated and can spread infectious disease agents. Therefore, all surfaces must be properly sanitized.

- Respiratory tract secretions may contaminate surfaces because they may contain viruses that remain infectious for varying periods of time, making it possible to acquire an infection by touching these surfaces.
- Walls, ceilings, floors, furnishings, equipment, and other surfaces should be maintained in good repair, free from visible soil, and in a clean condition.
- All surfaces, furnishings, and equipment that are not in good repair or have been contaminated by body fluids should not be used until repaired, cleaned, and, if need be, sanitized effectively.

- Tables used for play often are the same as those used for meals and snacks; therefore, cleaning/sanitizing these tables may reduce the risk of transmitting disease.
- Carpets, porous fabrics, other surfaces that trap soil, and potentially contaminated materials are not to be used in toilet rooms, diaper changing areas, and food preparation areas.
- Use caution when shampooing rugs used by children who are crawling. Cleaning with potentially hazardous chemicals should be scheduled to minimize exposure to children.

One way to measure compliance with the standard for cleanliness is to wipe a surface with a clean mop or rag and then insert the mop or rag in cold rinse water. If the surface is clean, no residue will appear in the rinse water.

Cleaning Equipment

- Only utility gloves/equipment designated for cleaning and sanitizing toilets should be used. After each use, utility gloves are to be washed with soapy water and dried.
  - ~ Disposable gloves commonly are made of latex or vinyl. If individuals sensitive to latex are present in the facility, only vinyl disposable gloves should be used.
- Disposable towels are preferred for cleaning and should be placed in a plastic-lined container until removed to outside garbage.
- After each day of use, cloth rags are to be placed in a closed, foot-operated receptacle until laundered.
- Reusable rags should be cleaned and sanitized before and after each day of use.
- Sponges are not recommended because they retain organic material that promotes bacterial growth.
- Mops should be assumed to be contaminated because they are used to remove contamination from floors and other soiled surfaces. Be sure they are cleaned and sanitized before and after a day of use.
  - ~ Bleach solution used for sanitizing the child care and school environment (see "Routine Cleaning, Sanitizing, and Disinfecting of Contaminated Surfaces" on page 15) can be used for sanitizing mops and rags. Detachable mop heads and reusable rags may be cleaned in a washing machine without other types of articles in the same load and dried in a mechanical dryer or hung to dry.

Waste Receptacles

Waste receptacles in toilet rooms should be kept clean, lined with plastic bags, in good repair, and emptied daily. Those that receive materials that are contaminated with body fluids should be of the hands-free type, such as a foot-operated receptacle. All other waste receptacles should be kept clean and emptied daily. This practice prevents the spread of disease.

Shoes

Infants put their hands in their mouths after touching play surfaces; therefore

- Shoes worn either outside of the infant play area or on surfaces contaminated with disease-causing agents may transfer infectious material to the infant play area.
- Shoes worn in toilet or diaper changing areas, play areas of other groups of children, and outdoors should not be allowed in the infant play area.
- Shoes/slippers worn only in the infant play area are allowed.
- As long as their feet are clean and have no sores or warts, children and adults may be barefoot in the play area.

Toys

- All toys can spread disease when children mouth or touch them after putting their hands in their mouths during play or eating or after toileting with inadequate hand washing.
- Toys that cannot be washed and sanitized should not be used.
- Mouthed toys or toys contaminated by body secretions or excretions should be removed from the play area until they are washed with water and detergent, rinsed, sanitized, and air-dried.
- Machine-washable cloth toys should be used only by one child until these toys are laundered.
- Indoor toys should not be shared between groups of infants or toddlers unless they are washed/sanitized before being moved from one group to another.
- Small, hard-surfaced toys can be cleaned in a dish pan labeled "soiled toys" containing soapy water to remove soil or a dry container used to bring the soiled toys to a toy cleaning area later in the day. A dishwasher that can sanitize dishes can be used to clean and sanitize hard-surfaced toys.
- Have more than one set of toys on hand so that one set can be used while the other is cleaned.

Mouthed Objects

Thermometers, pacifiers, teething toys, and similar objects should be cleaned and reusable parts should be sanitized between uses. Pacifiers should not be shared. Pacifiers should be cleaned and sanitized daily.

Bedding, Personal Clothing, and Cribs

Sleep equipment should be used only by one child, cleaned and sanitized before use by another child, and stored separately from others.

- Cribs and crib mattresses shall have a nonporous, easy-to-wipe surface.
- Bedding (eg, sheets, pillows, blankets, sleeping bags) should be washable.

• Lice infestation, scabies, and ringworm are among the most common contagious diseases in child care and school settings. Diseases can spread if bedding materials, jackets with hoods, and hats used by various children are stored so that they touch each other.

Potty Chairs and Toilets

• Potty chair use is not recommended and should be discouraged.
• If potty chairs are used, they should be
  ~ Made with a surface that is easily cleaned and sanitized.
  ~ Used only in a bathroom area.
  ~ Used over a surface that won't be damaged by moisture.
  ~ Out of reach of toilets or other potty chairs.
  ~ Emptied into a toilet, then cleaned in a sink that is used only for cleaning and sanitizing potty chairs.
• Toilets should be kept visibly clean and separate from the children's activity area.

Staff Training

Provide training for staff responsible for cleaning, including
• How to handle, mix, and store cleaning solutions (See "Sanitation, Disinfection, and Maintenance" on page 15.)
• Proper use of protective barriers (eg, gloves)
• Proper handling and disposal of contaminated materials
• Information required by the US Occupational Safety and Health Administration about the use of any chemical agents

Even if custodial services are provided under a contract with an outside service organization, be sure that an assigned staff member supervises routine cleaning of the facility according to the facility's schedule.

Hand Washing Steps

Because many infected people carry communicable diseases without having symptoms and are contagious before they experience symptoms, caregivers/teachers need to protect themselves and the children they serve by carrying out hygienic procedures on a routine basis.

Why Is Hand Washing Important?

Hand washing is the most effective means of reducing germs and infections in group care settings. Studies have shown that unwashed or improperly washed hands are primary carriers of infections. Lack of hand washing and poor hand washing techniques have contributed to many outbreaks of diarrhea among children and staff in group care settings. Conversely, adherence to good hand washing techniques has consistently demonstrated a reduction in disease transmission in child care and school settings. While working with children, caregivers/ teachers should not wear elaborate jewelry or long or artificial nails because these interfere with effective hand washing. Using hand lotion after hand washing to prevent chapping and cracking of skin also is important.

When to Wash Hands

To prevent the spread of infection, signs should be posted at each sink indicating when and how staff, volunteers, and children should wash their hands.

Hand washing should occur
• When arriving for the day or when moving from one group of children to another
• Before and after
  ~ Eating, handling food, or feeding a child; especially important for children who eat with their hands to decrease the amount of saliva (which may contain organisms) on their hands
  ~ Administering a medication
  ~ Playing with water that is used by more than one person
• After
  ~ Diapering and toileting
  ~ Handling body fluids (eg, mucus, blood, vomit)
  ~ Wiping noses, mouths, and sores
  ~ Handling uncooked food, especially raw meat and poultry
  ~ Handling pets and other animals
  ~ Playing in sandboxes (to prevent the ingestion of zoonotic parasites that could be present in contaminated sand and soil)
  ~ Cleaning
  ~ Handling garbage
• When leaving for the day

How to Wash Hands

Children and staff should wash hands using the following method:
• Make sure a clean, disposable paper (or single-use) towel is available.
• Turn on water (no less than 60°F and no more than 120°F).
• Moisten hands with water and apply liquid soap to hands.
• Rub hands together vigorously until soapy lather appears and continue for at least 10 seconds; rub areas between fingers, around nail beds, under fingernails and jewelry, and on back of hands.
• Rinse hands under running water until free of soap and dirt. Leave water running while drying hands.
• Dry hands with a clean, disposable paper towel or single-use cloth towel.
• If taps do not turn off automatically, turn taps off with a disposable paper towel or single-use cloth towel.
  ~ Shared towels can transmit infectious diseases.

- To dispose of towels
  - ~ Throw disposable towel in lined trash container.
  - ~ Place single-use cloth towel in laundry hamper.
  - ~ Hang individually labeled cloth towels to dry.
- If desired, use hand lotion from a liquid lotion dispenser to prevent chapping.

Running water over hands
- Removes soil, including infection-causing germs.
- Helps to create a lather to help loosen soil before applying soap.
- Helps soap lather loosen soil, making it easier to rinse from the skin.
- Rinses the lather off, removing the soil from the hands. Use warm water, no less than 60°F and no more than 120°F.
- Promotes adequate rinsing during hand washing. Use warm water if more comfortable than cold water.

Children and staff should use liquid soap because
- Although adequately drained bar soap has not been shown to transmit bacteria, bar soaps sitting in water have been shown to be heavily contaminated with *Pseudomonas* and other bacteria.
- Many children do not have the dexterity to handle a bar of soap, and many adults do not take the time to rinse the soil off before putting down the bar of soap.

Additional information
- Premoistened cleansing towelettes
  - ~ Do not effectively clean hands.
  - ~ May be used when running water is not available (eg, during an outing).
  - ~ May be used while in the middle of diapering. After removing the soiled diaper and before putting on a clean diaper, the caregiver's/teacher's hands (and often the child's hands, too) may come in contact with feces or urine by touching the soiled skin in the diaper area. Stepping away from the diaper table to wash hands at a sink at this point is not practical. Using a wipe to reduce the level of soil on the caregiver's/teacher's and child's hands at this point is a reasonable compromise.
- Antibacterial soaps may be used, but are neither required nor recommended.

Assisting Children With Hand Washing

Encouraging and teaching children good hand washing practices must be done in a safe manner. Washing infants' hands helps to reduce the spread of infection. Washing under water is best. Staff should wash their own hands after assisting children with hand washing.

Caregivers/teachers should provide assistance
- At a sink for infants who can be safely cradled in one arm
- For children who can stand, but not wash hands by themselves

For the child unable to stand and too heavy to hold at the sink to wash hands under running water, the following method should be used:
- Wipe child's hands with a damp paper towel moistened with a drop of liquid soap and discard towel.
- Wipe child's hands with a clean, wet paper towel until hands are free of soap and discard towel.
- Dry child's hands with a clean paper towel.

Using Alcohol-based Hand Rubs

The use of alcohol-based hand rub products (eg, liquid, gel, or foam hand sanitizers) does not substitute for hand washing in the group care setting. Caregivers/teachers should
- Limit the use of alcohol-based hand rubs to areas of the facility that are inaccessible to children (eg, in a kitchen that is off-limits to children or the maintenance equipment area). These products should not be accessible to children.
- Discourage alcohol-based hand rubs for hand hygiene in child-use areas. If used, they should be limited to situations in which there is no visible soil on the hands, sinks are not available, and the use and control of containers of the chemical sanitizer can ensure that no child can have independent use of the container or dispenser.
- Be sure that hand hygiene using alcohol-based hand rubs conforms to the manufacturer's instructions. The procedure for using alcohol-based rubs should include
  - ~ Applying the required volume of the product to the palm of one hand and rubbing together, covering all surfaces of the hands and fingers until the hands are dry. The required volume should keep the hand surfaces wet for at least 15 seconds or longer if so indicated by the manufacturer.
  - ~ Checking the dispenser systems for hand hygiene rubs on a regular schedule to be sure they deliver the required volume of the product and do not become clogged or malfunction in some other way.
  - ~ Storing supplies of alcohol-based hand rubs in cabinets or areas approved for flammable materials.
- Monitor hand hygiene with unannounced and regular direct observation. When hand rubs are used, check how much of the product is being used to be sure the appropriate amount gets used as a way to verify the staff who are authorized to use this method of hand hygiene are continuing to use the material as they should.

Diaper Changing Steps

The procedure for diaper changing is designed to reduce surface contamination that later will come in contact with uncontaminated surfaces such as hands, furnishings, and floors. Posting this multistep procedure may help caregivers/teachers routinely follow the correct steps to changing a child's diaper.

All staff should follow these diapering procedures.

Step 1: Get organized.

Before bringing child to diaper area, wash hands and gather the needed supplies.

- Nonabsorbent paper liner to cover changing surface from the child's shoulders to beyond the child's feet
- Fresh diaper
- Clean clothes (if needed)
- Wipes for cleaning child's bottom and wiping the caregiver's/teacher's and child's hands between taking off the soiled diaper and putting on the clean diaper
- Plastic bag for soiled clothes
- Disposable gloves (If used, put on before touching soiled clothing or diapers and remove before touching clean diapers and surfaces.)
- Thick application of any diaper cream (when appropriate) removed from container to a piece of disposable material (eg, tissue)

Step 2: Carry child to changing table, avoiding contact with soiled clothing.

- Always keep a hand on the child.
- If the child's feet cannot be kept out of the diaper or from contact with soiled skin during the changing process, remove child's shoes and socks so the child does not contaminate them with stool or urine.
- Put soiled clothes in a plastic bag and securely tie the bag to send the soiled clothes home.

Step 3: Clean the child's diaper area.

- Place the child on the diaper changing surface and unfasten the diaper but leave the soiled diaper under the child.
- If safety pins are used, close each pin immediately once it is removed and keep pins out of the child's reach (never hold pins in your mouth).
- Lift the child's legs as needed to use disposable wipes to clean the skin on the child's genitalia and buttocks.
- Remove stool and urine from front to back and use a fresh wipe each time.
- Put the soiled wipes in the soiled diaper or directly into a plastic-lined, covered, foot-operated receptacle.

Step 4: Remove the soiled diaper without contaminating any surface not already in contact with stool or urine.

- Fold the soiled surface inward.
- Put soiled disposable diapers in a plastic-lined, covered, foot-operated receptacle. If reusable cloth diapers are used, put the soiled cloth diaper (without emptying or rinsing) in a plastic bag or into a plastic-lined, covered, foot-operated receptacle to give to parents or laundry service.
- If gloves were used, remove them and put them into a plastic-lined, covered, foot-operated receptacle.
- Whether or not gloves were used, use a disposable wipe to clean the surfaces of the caregiver's/teacher's hands and another to clean the child's hands and put the wipes into the plastic-lined, hands-free covered can.
- Check for spills under the child. If there are any, use the paper that extends under the child's feet to fold over the disposable paper so a fresh, unsoiled paper surface is now under the child's buttocks.

Step 5: Put on a clean diaper and dress the child.

- Slide a fresh diaper under the child.
- Use tissue to apply any necessary diaper creams, discarding the tissue in a plastic-lined, covered, foot-operated receptacle.
- Observe, note, and plan to report any skin problems such as redness, skin cracks, or bleeding.
- Fasten the diaper (if pins are used, place your hand between the child and diaper when inserting the pin) and reclothe the child.

Step 6: Wash the child's hands and return the child to a supervised area.

- Use soap and water (no less than 60°F and no more than 120°F) to wash the child's hands.
- If a child is too heavy to hold or cannot stand at the sink, use the following method to wash hands:
  ~ Wipe the child's hands with a damp paper towel moistened with a drop of liquid soap.
  ~ Wipe the child's hands with a paper towel wet with clean water.
  ~ Dry the child's hands with a paper towel.

Step 7: Clean and sanitize the diaper changing surface.

- Dispose of the paper liner used on the diaper changing surface in a plastic-lined, covered, foot-operated receptacle.
- Clean any visible soil from the changing surface with detergent and water; rinse with water.

- Spray a sanitizing bleach solution onto the entire changing surface (see "Sanitation, Disinfection, and Maintenance" on page 15).
- Leave the bleach sanitizer on the surface for at least 2 minutes (the surface can be wiped dry or left to air-dry).

Step 8: Wash your hands and record the diaper change in the child's daily log.
- Wash hands using soap and water, using a paper towel to turn off water faucet.
- In the daily log, record what was in the diaper and any problems (eg, diarrhea, unusual color or odor, blood in the stool, any skin irritation).

The procedure for diaper changing is designed to
- Reduce surface contamination with uncontaminated surfaces (eg, hands, furnishings).
- Ensure the child's safety by assembling supplies before bringing child to the changing area.
- Reduce possible contamination and spreading of disease by taking supplies directly from their containers and leaving containers in their assigned areas.

Remember
- Food preparation should not be permitted in the diapering area.
- Gloves are not necessary but may reduce contamination of hands and infectious agents under the fingernails.
- After diapering, clean visible soil from surface with detergent followed by bleach solution, which should be left on for 2 minutes, then wiped or air-dried (see "Sanitation, Disinfection, and Maintenance" on page 15).

Components of a Diapering Area
Diaper changing areas should
- Not be located in food preparation areas.
- Not be used for temporary placement of food or utensils.
- Be conveniently located, washable, and lined with plastic.
- Have tightly covered, hands-free receptacles nearby to prevent environmental contamination so children do not come in contact with disease-bearing body fluids.
- Be positioned to allow caregivers/teachers to maintain constant sight and sound supervision of children.
- Be designed to prevent contamination during the diaper changing process.

Diaper Changing Tables
- There should be one diaper changing table per infant or toddler group to
  ~ Allow sufficient time for changing diapers.
  ~ Allow for cleaning and sanitizing between use.
- It should be used only by those children in each group.
- Tables and sinks should not be used by more than one group because
  ~ Diaper changing and cleaning/changing surfaces takes time.
  ~ Disease spreads more easily when caregivers/teachers from different groups use the same diaper changing surface.
- Diaper changing tables and sinks should not be placed between 2 classrooms (commingling of 2 groups) to reduce possible cross-contamination.

Changing Table Requirements
Changing tables should be
- Made of moisture-proof, nonabsorbent, smooth surfaces that do not trap soil and are easily sanitized
- Sturdy
- At a convenient height (between 28" and 32" high) for use by caregivers/teachers
- Be equipped with railings or barriers that extend at least 6" above the change surface

These requirements are designed to prevent disease transmission and accidental falls and provide safety during diapering.

Sinks in Diaper Changing Areas
- Sinks in diaper changing areas should be within arm's reach of the caregivers/teachers to avoid transfer of contaminants to other surfaces.
- At least one sink should be available for every 2 changing tables.
- Sinks and diaper changing tables should be assigned to a specific group of children.
- Sinks should not be used for bathing or removing smeared fecal material.
- Drinking utensils and food should not be washed in these sinks.

Caregiver/Teacher Health

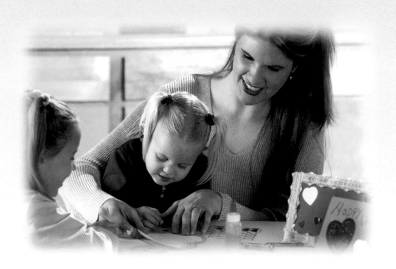

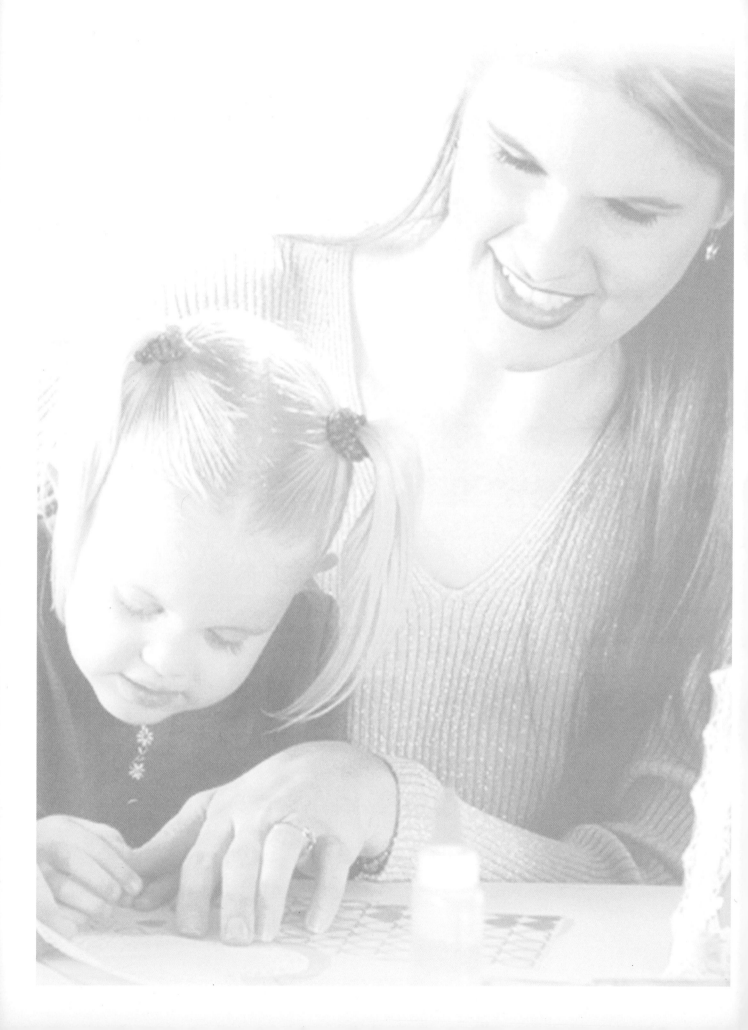

Caregiver/Teacher Health

Introduction

Caregiver/teacher health is very important in maintaining a successful and healthy environment. A daily evaluation of each staff member, substitute, and volunteer for obvious signs of ill health by an administrator or other assigned caregiver/teacher is important. These informal checks should be part of each day's routine greeting as each person comes into the facility.

Adults who care for children should
• Be healthy and able to perform the duties required of them.
• Have regular health checkups.
• Have up-to-date immunizations, including receipt of an annual influenza vaccine.
• Take appropriate precautions to minimize the exposure of others to infections and illnesses.

Health Appraisals

Adults who care for children and work more than 40 hours per month are required to have
• A preemployment health appraisal (health history review, physical examinations, screening tests, and professional evaluation of results)
• Additional health appraisals every 2 years
• Documentation on file that the individual's health appraisals included
    ~ Health history
    ~ Physical and dental examinations
    ~ Vision and hearing screening
    ~ A preemployment tuberculosis (TB) screening test (using the Mantoux test, 1- or 2-step procedure) with follow-up of any positive results
        ❖ The 2-step process is used in those who may have a diminished immune response.
        ❖ If the result of a first skin test is negative, the test is repeated again in a month or so to "boost" the stimulation of the test material to see whether the first test gave a false-negative result.
        ❖ Tuberculosis screening should be a 2-step process for those older than 60 years.
    ~ Up-to-date immunization or certified immune status to measles, mumps, rubella, diphtheria, tetanus, polio, varicella, influenza, and hepatitis B and evaluation of risk-related need for hepatitis A and pneumococcal polysaccharide vaccines
    ~ Assessment of risk from exposure to common childhood infections (eg, parvovirus, cytomegalovirus, chickenpox) as determined by the adult's health professional

    ~ Assessment and description of job-related health concerns (eg, orthopedic, psychologic, neurologic, sensory limitations, communicable diseases that require accommodations to complete daily tasks)

All high-risk adults who reside in a family child care home and any adult who works with children (even less than 40 hours a week) must complete TB screening. Adults at high risk for TB include those who are foreign born, have a history of homelessness, are human immunodeficiency virus (HIV) infected, have contact with a prison population, have traveled to a country where TB is endemic, or have contact with someone who has active TB. After the initial TB screening, routine annual screening should be limited to those whose activities continue to place them at high risk for exposure to TB. All adults who work in group care settings should be encouraged to have a full health appraisal as well.

Health Limitations of Staff

Staff and volunteers must have a licensed health professional's release to return to work when
• The program has any concern that the adult may have a harmful communicable disease (eg, reportable to the health department; see table on page 30 for some examples) or because of continuing symptoms or unclear information about the status of the adult.
• They experience a condition that may affect their ability to do their jobs.
• They require accommodations to prevent illness or injury in their work.
• They return after a serious or prolonged illness or after a job-related injury.
• Their condition or health could affect assignment to a new role in the child care program or school.
• There are insurance issues or liability risks for the child care program or school related to their health problem.

Infectious Diseases

Adults who work in group care settings are at increased risk for acquiring and spreading infectious diseases. Caregivers/teachers are in constant contact with nasal and oral secretions of children. Early in the course of an infectious illness, even before children seem ill, these secretions carry enough germs to cause disease in others. Especially during the first year or so of contact with young children, adults who work in child care programs or schools may have more symptomatic illnesses than those who do not work with children. Usually the frequency of infectious illness becomes less after a while, as the adults develop immunity. Staff sick leave is important because it

- May minimize the spread of harmful communicable diseases (see table on page 30)
- May promote full recovery from illness, which may improve resistance to the next exposure to infection and improve job performance

Staff who are ill or who become ill during the day should be allowed and encouraged to go home. However, it is understandable that they may be reluctant to go home because of the potential loss of income or difficulties in arranging for a substitute caregiver/teacher. Advance planning for substitutes and authorized, paid sick leave can help.

Staff should immediately report to their supervisor any signs of infection or illness that may affect the health or safety of children or adults. Clear and open communication about illness can help to

- Identify potential health risks.
- Prevent the spread of harmful infections and illnesses.

Dental Decay

Early childhood caries (dental decay)

- Is a disease that is mostly preventable
- Is an infectious disease because bacteria, which are partially responsible for the decay, can be transmitted from a parent or an adult caregiver/teacher to children
- Occurs in all racial and socioeconomic groups, but those from low-income families are at an increased risk

Adults with active tooth decay are more likely to transmit bacteria to children in their care and should

- Brush thoroughly twice daily and floss once each day.
- Have dental care to correct their tooth decay and infectious status.
- Use careful and frequent hand washing.
- Not share utensils or clean pacifiers with their saliva.

For more information, visit www.aap.org and search for "oral health."

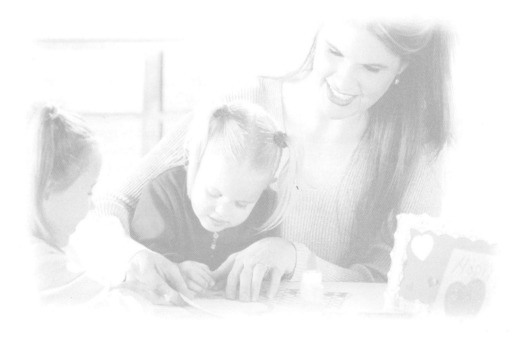

CHAPTER 5

Recognizing the Ill Child: Inclusion/ Exclusion Criteria

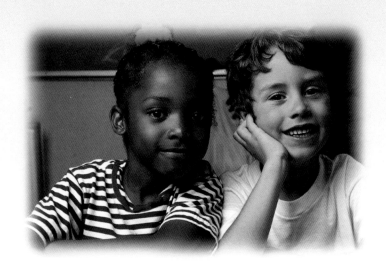

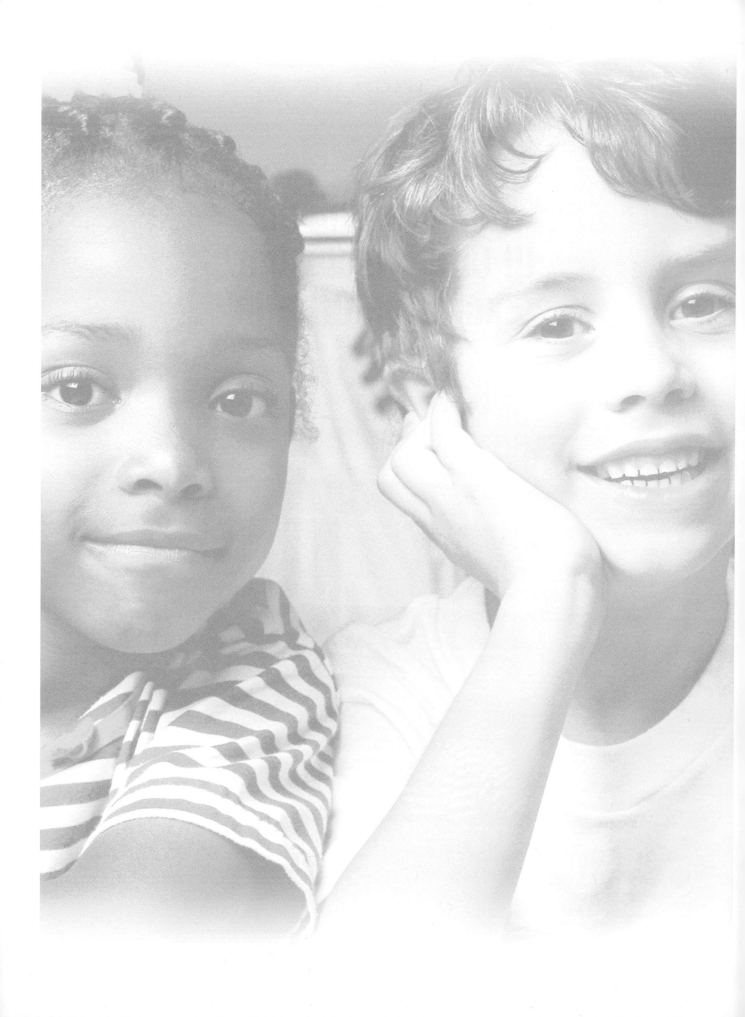

Recognizing the Ill Child: Inclusion/Exclusion Criteria

Daily Health Assessment Check

The staff of a child care program or school who are familiar with the behavior and appearance of the enrolled children should assess each child's health status when the child arrives and periodically throughout the day. This assessment involves observing the child, speaking with parents, and, if applicable, talking with the child.

Staff should be instructed to observe and document

- Changes in behavior or appearance
- Any skin rashes and itchy skin or scalp
- Signs of fever such as flushed appearance or shivering (Daily temperature monitoring, in the absence of behavior change, is not recommended.)
- Complaints of pain or not feeling well
- Vomiting, diarrhea, and drainage from eye(s)
- When a child or family member has been exposed to a harmful communicable disease

Sharing this information among caregivers/teachers and families helps everyone to be on the lookout for signs and symptoms of illness and discuss the implication of potential exposure to illness with health professionals.

When to Get Immediate Medical Help

- Call emergency medical services (usually 911) for the child who
  - ~ Has difficulty breathing or is unable to speak
  - ~ Has blue, purple, or gray skin or lips
  - ~ Is unconscious
  - ~ Is vomiting blood
  - ~ Has a stiff neck with headache and fever
  - ~ Is severely dehydrated with sunken eyes, lethargy, and no tears and not urinating
  - ~ Has had a serious injury or has severe pain
  - ~ Is increasingly less responsive
  - ~ Is acting strangely, much less alert, or much more withdrawn than usual
- Get medical attention within 1 hour for the child who
  - ~ Has a fever and who looks more than mildly ill
  - ~ Is younger than 2 months with a temperature above 100°F axillary (armpit) or 101°F rectally
  - ~ Has a quickly spreading purple or red rash
  - ~ Has a large volume of blood in the stools
  - ~ Has an injury that may require medical treatment such as a cut that may require stitches
  - ~ Has an animal bite that breaks the skin
  - ~ Has any medical condition that is outlined in the child's care plan as requiring medical attention

Children Who Are Ill

When a child becomes ill but does not require immediate medical help, a determination must be made whether the child requires exclusion. Most illnesses do not require exclusion. The caregiver/teacher should determine if the

- Illness prevents the child from participating comfortably in activities.
- Illness results in a need for care that is greater than the staff can provide without compromising the health and safety of other children.
- Illness poses a risk of spread of disease to others.

If any of these criteria is met, the child should be excluded, regardless of the type of illness.

Conditions That Do Not Require Exclusion

- Common colds, runny noses (regardless of color or consistency of nasal discharge), and coughs.
- Fever without any signs or symptoms of illness in children who are older than 4 months. For this purpose, fever is defined as temperature above 101°F orally, above 102°F rectally, or 100°F or higher taken axillary (armpit) or measured by any equivalent method. Fever is an indication of the body's response to something, but is neither a disease nor a serious problem by itself. Body temperature can be elevated by overheating caused by overdressing or a hot environment, reactions to medications, and response to infection. If the child is behaving normally but has a fever, the cause of the fever should be sought, but the child does not require exclusion for fever alone.
- Watery eye discharge without fever, eye pain, or eyelid redness.
- Yellow or white eye drainage that is not associated with pink or red conjunctiva (ie, the whites of the eyes).
- Rash without fever and behavioral changes.
- Lice or nits without lice (may delay treatment until the end of the day).
- Ringworm (may delay treatment until the end of the day).
- Thrush (ie, white spots or patches in the mouth).
- Fifth disease (slapped cheek disease, parvovirus B19) in a child without immune problems.
- Cytomegalovirus infection.
- Chronic hepatitis B virus infection.
- Human immunodeficiency virus (HIV) infection, with consideration of risk to the HIV-infected child or others decided on a case-by-case basis by health professionals.

• The presence of infectious germs in stool or urine without illness symptoms (exceptions include potentially serious organisms [eg, *Escherichia coli* O157:H7, *Shigella*, *Salmonella typhi*]). Children with *E coli* O157:H7 or *Shigella* must be excluded until 2 stool cultures are negative and the child is cleared to return by local health department officials. Children with *S typhi* must be excluded until 3 stool cultures are negative and they are cleared by a health professional or local health department officials.

• Children with chronic infectious conditions that can be accommodated in the program according to the legal requirements of federal law in the Americans with Disabilities Act (eg, HIV infection). The act requires that child care programs and schools make reasonable accommodations for children with disabilities and/or chronic illnesses, considering each child individually.

Conditions Requiring Temporary Exclusion

Temporary exclusion is recommended when

• The illness prevents the child from participating comfortably in activities as determined by the staff of the child care program or school.

• The illness results in a greater need for care than the staff of the program determine they can provide without compromising their ability to care for other children.

• The child has any of the following conditions, unless a health professional determines the child's condition does not require exclusion:

~ Appears to be severely ill.

~ Fever (temperature above 101°F orally, above 102°F rectally, or 100°F or higher taken axillary [armpit] or measured by an equivalent method) *and* behavior change or other signs and symptoms (eg, sore throat, rash, vomiting, diarrhea). An unexplained temperature above 100°F axillary (armpit) or 101°F rectally in a child younger than 4 months should be medically evaluated. For example, an infant with a fever but behaving normally on the day after an immunization that is known to sometimes cause fever does not require exclusion. (Exception: *Any infant younger than 2 months with a fever should get medical attention within an hour.*) When taking temperature, remember

❖ The amount of temperature elevation varies at different body sites.

❖ The height of fever does not indicate a more or less severe illness.

❖ The method chosen to take a child's temperature depends on the need for accuracy, available equipment, the skill of the person taking the temperature, and the ability of the child to assist in the procedure.

❖ Oral temperatures are not usually reliable for children younger than 4 years.

❖ Rectal temperatures should be taken only by persons with specific health training in performing this procedure.

❖ Axillary (armpit) temperatures are only accurate in young infants.

❖ Electronic devices for measuring temperature in the ear canal or skin over the temple (next to the eye) may not be reliable or accurate ways of measuring temperature. At their best, they give temperatures that are similar to rectal temperature. These devices require periodic calibration and those using them should receive specific training to be sure they are used correctly.

~ Diarrhea—defined by more watery stools, decreased form of stool that is not associated with changes of diet, and increased frequency of passing stool that is not contained by the child's ability to use the toilet—until the diarrhea resolves. Exceptions include

❖ Toxin-producing *E coli* or *Shigella* infection: until the diarrhea resolves and the test results of 2 stool cultures are negative for these organisms.

❖ *S typhi* infection: until the diarrhea resolves, the test results of 3 stool cultures are negative for these organisms, and the child has been cleared by a health professional or health department.

~ Blood in the stools not explained by dietary change, medication, or hard stools.

~ Vomiting more than 2 times in the previous 24 hours, unless the vomiting is determined to be caused by a noncommunicable condition and the child is not in danger of dehydration.

~ Abdominal pain that continues for more than 2 hours or intermittent pain associated with fever or other signs or symptoms.

~ Mouth sores with drooling.

~ Rash with fever or behavioral changes.

~ Pink or red conjunctiva (ie, whites of the eyes) with white or yellow eye mucus drainage (signs of bacterial infection), often with matted eyelids after sleep and eye pain, or redness of the eyelids or skin around the eye until treatment has been started (viral conjunctivitis usually has a clear, watery discharge that may not require exclusion).

~ Tuberculosis, until the child's physician or local health department states child is on appropriate treatment and can return.

~ Impetigo, until 24 hours after treatment has been started.

~ Streptococcal pharyngitis (ie, strep throat or other streptococcal infection), until 24 hours after treatment has been started.

~ Head lice or nits, until after the first treatment (note: exclusion is not necessary before the end of the program day).

~ Scabies, until after treatment has been given.

~ Chickenpox (varicella) until all lesions have dried or crusted (usually 6 days after onset of rash).

~ Pertussis, until 5 days of appropriate antibiotic treatment.

~ Mumps, until 9 days after onset of parotid gland swelling.

~ Measles, until 4 days after onset of rash.

~ Hepatitis A virus infection, until 1 week after onset of illness or jaundice or as directed by the health department when immune globulin has been given to the appropriate children and adult contacts.

~ Any child determined by the local health department to be contributing to the transmission of illness during an outbreak.

For more details and other diseases, see Chapter 6, "Signs and Symptoms Chart," on page 31.

Procedures for a Child Who Requires Exclusion

The caregiver/teacher will

- Provide care for the child in a place where the child will be comfortable and supervised by someone who knows the child well and will continue to observe the child for new or worsening symptoms.
- Ask the family to pick up the child as soon as possible.
- Ask the family to relay the advice received from the health professional, if a medical visit is deemed necessary.
- Follow the advice of the child's health professional.
- Contact the local health department if there is a question of a reportable (harmful) communicable disease. If there are conflicting opinions from different health professionals about the management of a child with a reportable communicable disease, the health department has the legal authority to make a final determination.
- Document actions in the child's file with date, time, symptoms, and actions taken (and by whom); sign and date the document.
- Sanitize toys and other items the child may have put in his or her mouth and continue to practice good hand washing techniques.

Reportable Conditions

The infectious diseases designated as notifiable in the United States at the national level by the Centers for Disease Control and Prevention (as of 2004) are listed in the table on page 30.

The caregiver/teacher should contact the local health department

- When a child or staff member who is in contact with others has a reportable disease
- If a reportable illness occurs among the staff, children, or families involved with the program
- For assistance in managing a suspected outbreak

Caregivers/teachers should work with their health consultants to develop policies and procedures for alerting staff and families about their responsibility to report illnesses to the program and for the program to report diseases to the local health authorities.

Preparing for Managing Illness

Caregivers/teachers should

- Prepare families for inevitable illnesses ahead of time.
- Review with families the inclusion/exclusion criteria and that the program staff (not the families) make the final decision about whether ill children whose families want them to participate may stay based on the inclusion/exclusion criteria.
- Develop, with a health consultant, protocols and procedures for handling children's illnesses, including care plans and an inclusion/exclusion policy.
- Only ask for a health professional's note to readmit if professional advice is needed to determine whether the child is a health risk to others or the child needs special care.
- Rely on the family's description of the child's behavior to determine whether the child is well enough to return, unless the child's status is unclear from the family's report.

Infectious Diseases Designated as Notifiable at the National Level—United States, 2004

Acquired immunodeficiency syndrome
(AIDS)
Anthrax
Botulism
Botulism, foodborne
Botulism, infant
Botulism, other (wound & unspecified)
Brucellosis
Chancroid
Chlamydia trachomatis, genital infections
Cholera
Coccidioidomycosis
Cryptosporidiosis
Cyclosporiasis
Diphtheria
Ehrlichiosis
Ehrlichiosis, human granulocytic
Ehrlichiosis, human monocytic
Ehrlichiosis, human, other or
unspecified agent
Encephalitis/meningitis, arboviral
Encephalitis/meningitis, California
serogroup viral
Encephalitis/meningitis, eastern equine
Encephalitis/meningitis, Powassan
Encephalitis/meningitis, St Louis
Encephalitis/meningitis, western equine
Encephalitis/meningitis, West Nile
Enterohemorrhagic *Escherichia coli*
Enterohemorrhagic *Escherichia coli,*
O157:H7
Enterohemorrhagic *Escherichia coli,* shiga
toxin positive, serogroup non-O157
Enterohemorrhagic *Escherichia coli* shiga
toxin+ (not serogrouped)
Giardiasis

Gonorrhea
Haemophilus influenzae, invasive disease
Hansen disease (leprosy)
Hantavirus pulmonary syndrome
Hemolytic uremic syndrome, post-diarrheal
Hepatitis, viral, acute
Hepatitis A, acute
Hepatitis B, acute
Hepatitis B virus, perinatal infection
Hepatitis C, acute
Hepatitis, viral, chronic
Chronic hepatitis B
Hepatitis C virus infection (past or
present)
Human immunodeficiency virus (HIV)
infection
HIV infection, adult (≥13 years)
HIV infection, pediatric (<13 years)
Legionellosis
Listeriosis
Lyme disease
Malaria
Measles
Meningococcal disease
Mumps
Pertussis
Plague
Poliomyelitis, paralytic
Psittacosis
Q fever
Rabies
Rabies, animal
Rabies, human
Rocky Mountain spotted fever
Rubella
Rubella, congenital syndrome

Salmonellosis
Severe acute respiratory syndrome-
associated coronavirus (SARS-CoV)
disease
Shigellosis
Smallpox
Streptococcal disease, invasive, group A
Streptococcal toxic shock syndrome
Streptococcus pneumoniae, drug resistant,
invasive disease
Streptococcus pneumoniae, invasive in
children <5 years
Syphilis
Syphilis, primary
Syphilis, secondary
Syphilis, latent
Syphilis, early latent
Syphilis, late latent
Syphilis, latent, unknown duration
Neurosyphilis
Syphilis, late, non-neurological
Syphilis, congenital
Syphilitic stillbirth
Tetanus
Toxic shock syndrome
Trichinosis
Tuberculosis
Tularemia
Typhoid fever
Vancomycin—intermediate *Staphylococcus
aureus* (VISA)
Vancomycin—resistant *Staphylococcus
aureus* (VRSA)
Varicella (morbidity)
Varicella (deaths only)
Yellow fever

Epidemiology Program Office, Division of Public Health Surveillance and Informatics, Centers for Disease Control and Prevention. Nationally notifiable infectious diseases. United States 2004. Available at: http://www.cdc.gov/epo/dphsi/phs/infdis2004.htm. Accessed August 23, 2004

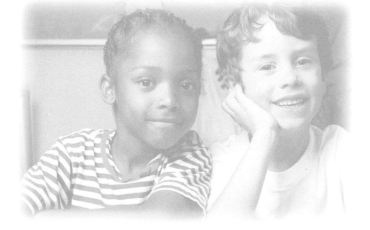

CHAPTER 6

Signs and Symptoms Chart

The following chart lists in alphabetic order some of the most common signs and symptoms that children in group care settings may develop when they have an infectious disease. Health professionals can use this chart to discuss with caregivers/teachers what they should look for to recognize diseases and make decisions about when children need medical care. Caregivers/teachers should use this information to be aware of what might cause various signs and symptoms, when it is appropriate to notify a health consultant and/or the parent, and the criteria to determine when children should be excluded from and can return to a group setting. Caregivers/teachers should work with health professionals to ensure an appropriate diagnosis and treatment.

Note that the chart indicates when visits to a health professional are necessary. Not all children who are excluded from a group care setting require a visit to a health professional prior to return to care. However, if you are concerned about the nature of the child's specific illness or need instructions about how to care for the child, the child's parent/guardian can make a phone call to the child's health professional to clarify whether further evaluation is necessary. With parent/guardian consent, the child's health professional can give additional instructions in writing or over the phone to caregivers/teachers.

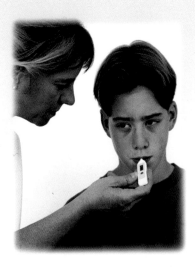

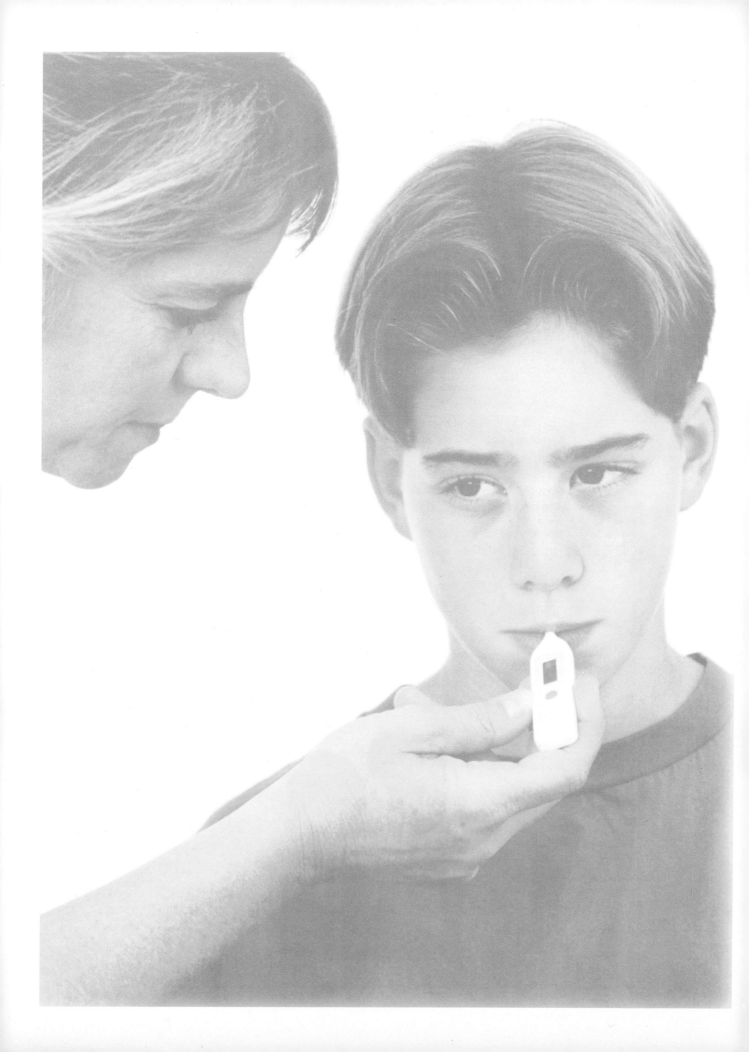

Signs and Symptoms Chart

Symptom	Common Causes	Complaints or What Might Be Seen	Notify Health Consultant	Notify Parent	Temporarily Exclude? (See also "When to Get Immediate Medical Help" on page 27).	If Excluded, Readmit When
Cold Symptoms	*Viruses* (early stage of many viruses) • Adenovirus • Coxsackievirus • Enterovirus • Parainfluenza virus • Respiratory syncytial virus • Rhinovirus • Coronavirus *Bacteria* • Mycoplasma	• Runny or stuffy nose • Scratchy throat • Coughing • Sneezing • Watery eyes • Fever		Yes	**No, unless** • Fever accompanied by behavior change. • Child looks or acts very ill. • Child has difficulty breathing. • Child has blood red or purple rash not associated with injury. • The child meets other exclusion criteria (see "Conditions Requiring Temporary Exclusion" on page 28).	• Exclusion criteria are resolved.
Cough (May come from congestion anywhere from ears to lungs. Cough is a body response to something that is irritating tissues in the airway.)	• Common cold • Lower respiratory infection (eg, pneumonia, bronchitis) • Croup • Bronchiolitis • Asthma • Sinus infection	• Dry or wet cough • Runny nose (clear, white, or yellow-green) • Sore throat • Throat irritation • Hoarse voice, barking cough		Yes	**No, unless** • Severe cough • Rapid and/or difficult breathing • Wheezing if not already evaluated and treated • Cyanosis (ie, blue color of skin and mucous membranes)	• Exclusion criteria are resolved.
Diaper Rash	• Irritation by rubbing of diaper material against skin wet with urine or stool • Infection with yeast or bacteria	• Redness • Scaling • Red bumps • Sores • Cracking of skin in diaper region		Yes	**No, unless** • Oozing sores that leak body fluids outside the diaper	• Exclusion criteria are resolved.

Symptom	Common Causes	Complaints or What Might Be Seen	Notify Health Consultant	Notify Parent	Temporarily Exclude? (See also "When to Get Immediate Medical Help" on page 27).	If Excluded, Readmit When
Diarrhea	Usually viral, less commonly bacterial or parasitic	• Frequent loose or watery stools compared to child's normal pattern (Note that exclusively breastfed infants normally have frequent unformed and somewhat watery stools, or may have several days with no stools.) • Abdominal cramps • Fever • Generally not feeling well • Sometimes accompanied by vomiting	• For one or more cases of bloody diarrhea or more than usual number of children with diarrhea in group	Yes	**Yes, if** • Diarrhea not contained in toilet (All infants with diarrhea must be excluded.) • Blood/mucus in stool • Abnormal color of stool for child (eg, all black or very pale) • No urine output in 8 hours • Jaundice (ie, yellow skin or eyes) • Fever with behavior change • Looks or acts very ill	• Cleared to return by health professional for all cases of bloody diarrhea and diarrhea caused by *Shigella*, *Salmonella*, or *Giardia*. • Stool is contained in toilet (for toilet-trained children). • Even if stools stay loose, the child is able to participate and the stool consistency has not changed for a week.
Difficult or Noisy Breathing	1. Common cold 2. Croup 3. Epiglottitis 4. Bronchiolitis 5. Asthma 6. Pneumonia 7. Object stuck in airway	1. Stuffy nose, sore throat, cough, and/or mild fever. 2 and 3. Barking cough, hoarseness, fever, possible chest discomfort (symptoms worse at night), and/or very noisy breathing, especially when breathing in. 3. Gasping noisily for breath with mouth wide open, chin pulled down, high fever, and/or bluish (cyanotic) nails and skin; drooling, unwilling to lie down.		Yes	**Yes, if** • Hard, fast, difficult breathing that does not improve with any medication the program has been instructed to use for this child's difficult breathing • Barking cough with fever or behavior change • Chest retractions • Breathing problem that makes feeding very difficult • Looks or acts very ill	• Cleared to return by health professional. • Exclusion criteria are resolved.

Symptom	Common Causes	Complaints or What Might Be Seen	Notify Health Consultant	Notify Parent	Temporarily Exclude? (See also "When to Get Immediate Medical Help" on page 27).	If Excluded, Readmit When
Difficult or Noisy Breathing, continued		4 and 5. Child is working hard to breathe; rapid breathing; space between ribs looks like it is sucked in with each breath (retractions); wheezing; whistling sound with breathing; cold/cough; irritable and unwell. Takes longer to breathe out than to breathe in. 6. Deep cough, fever, rapid breathing, or space between ribs looks like it is sucked in with each breath (retractions). 7. Symptoms similar to croup (2).		Yes		
Earache	• Bacteria or viruses • Often occurs in context of common cold	• Fever • Pain or irritability • Difficulty hearing • "Blocked ears" • Drainage • Swelling around ear		Yes	**No, unless** • Unable to participate. • Care would compromise staff's ability to care for other children. • Fever with behavior change. Note: Ear infections are not contagious. By the time a middle ear infection develops, the infection that causes the ear infection is much less contagious than in the days before the ear symptoms develop.	• Exclusion criteria are resolved.
Eye Irritation, Pinkeye	1. Bacterial infection of the membrane covering the eye and eyelid (bacterial conjunctivitis) 2. Viral infection of the membrane covering the eye and eyelid (viral conjunctivitis)	1. Pink color instead of whites of eyes *and* thick yellow/green discharge. May be irritated, swollen, or crusted in the morning.	Yes	Yes	*For bacterial conjunctivitis* **Yes** *For other forms* **No, unless** • The child meets other exclusion criteria (see "Conditions Requiring Temporary Exclusion" on page 28).	• *For bacterial conjunctivitis,* on medication at least 24 hours (if indicated). • Exclusion criteria are resolved.

Symptom	Common Causes	Complaints or What Might Be Seen	Notify Health Consultant	Notify Parent	Temporarily Exclude? (See also "When to Get Immediate Medical Help" on page 27).	If Excluded, Readmit When
Eye Irritation, Pinkeye, continued	3. Allergic irritation of the membrane covering the eye and eyelid (allergic conjunctivitis) 4. Chemical irritation of the membrane covering the eye and eyelid (irritant conjunctivitis) (eg, swimming in heavily chlorinated water, air pollution)	2. Pinkish/red, irritated, swollen eyes; watery discharge; possible upper respiratory infection. 3 and 4. Red, tearing, itchy eyes; runny nose, sneezing; watery discharge.			Note: One type of viral conjunctivitis spreads rapidly and requires exclusion. If more than 1 or 2 children in the group have watery red eyes without any known chemical irritant exposure, exclusion may be required and health authorities should be notified.	
Fever	• Any viral, bacterial, or parasitic infection • Overheating • Reaction to medication (eg, vaccine, oral)	Flushing, tired, irritable, decreased activity Notes • Fever alone is not harmful. When a child has an infection, raising the body temperature is part of the body's normal defense against outside attacks. • Rapid elevation of body temperature sometimes can trigger a febrile seizure in young children; this is usually outgrown by age 6 years. The first time a febrile seizure happens, the child requires evaluation. These seizures are frightening, but do not cause the child any long-term harm. Parents should inform their child's health professional every time the child has a seizure, even if the child is known to have febrile seizures.		Yes	**No, unless** • Behavior change. • Unable to participate. • Care would compromise staff's ability to care for other children. Note: Temperatures considered meaningfully elevated above normal, leading to concern of possible disease, for children older than 4 months are • 100°F axillary (armpit) • 101°F orally • 102°F rectally • Aural (ear) temperature equal to oral or rectal temperature ***Get immediate medical attention when*** infant younger than 4 months has an unexplained temperature of 101°F rectally or 100°F axillary. Any infant younger than 2 months with fever should get medical attention within an hour.	• Able to participate. • Exclusion criteria are resolved.

Symptom	Common Causes	Complaints or What Might Be Seen	Notify Health Consultant	Notify Parent	Temporarily Exclude? (See also "When to Get Immediate Medical Help" on page 27).	If Excluded, Readmit When
Fever, continued		**Warning:** *Do not* give aspirin to reduce a fever. Aspirin has been linked to an increased risk of Reye syndrome (a rare and serious disease affecting the brain and liver).				
Headache	• Any bacterial/viral infection • Other noninfectious causes	• Tired and irritable • Can occur with or without other symptoms		Yes	**No, unless** • Child is unable to participate. Note: **Notify health professional** in case of sudden, severe headache with vomiting or stiff neck that might signal meningitis. The stiff neck of concern is reluctance and unusual discomfort when the child is asked to look at her/his "belly button" (putting chin to chest)—different from soreness in the side of the neck.	• Able to participate
Itching	1. Ringworm 2. Chickenpox 3. Pinworm 4. Head lice 5. Scabies 6. Allergic or irritant reaction 7. Dry skin or eczema 8. Impetigo	1. Itchy ring-shaped patches on skin or bald patches on scalp. 2. Blister-like spots surrounded by red halos on scalp, face, and body; fever; irritable. 3. Anal itching. 4. Small insects or white egg sheaths (nits) in hair. 5. Severely itchy red bumps on warm areas of body, especially between fingers or toes. 6. Raised, large, circular, mobile rash; reddening of the skin; blisters.	• For infestations such as lice and scabies; if more than one child in group has impetigo or ringworm; for chickenpox	Yes	*For chickenpox, scabies, and impetigo* **Yes** *For ringworm and head lice* **Yes, at the end of the day** • Children should be referred to a health professional at the end of the day for treatment. *For pinworm, allergic or irritant reactions, and eczema* **No, unless** • Appears infected Note: Exclusion for hives is only necessary to obtain medical advice for care, if there is no previously made assessment and care plan for the hives.	• Seen and cleared by health professional • On medication at least 24 hours (if indicated)

Symptom	Common Causes	Complaints or What Might Be Seen	Notify Health Consultant	Notify Parent	Temporarily Exclude? (See also "When to Get Immediate Medical Help" on page 27).	If Excluded, Readmit When
Itching, continued		7. Dry areas on body. More often worse on cheeks, in front of elbows, and behind knees. In infants, may be dry areas on fronts of legs and anywhere else on body, but not usually in diaper area. If swollen, red, or oozing, think about infection. 8. Areas of crusted yellow, oozing sores. Often around mouth or nasal openings.				
Mouth Sores	1. Oral thrush (yeast infection) 2. Herpes or coxsackie-virus infection 3. Canker sores	1. White patches on tongue and along cheeks 2. Pain on swallowing; fever; painful, yellowish spots in mouth; swollen neck glands; fever blister, cold sore; reddened, swollen, painful lips 3. Painful ulcers on cheeks or gums		Yes	**No, unless** • Drooling steadily related to mouth sores. • Unable to participate. • Care would compromise staff's ability to care for other children.	• Able to participate. • Exclusion criteria are resolved.
Rash	Many causes 1. Viral: roseola infantum, fifth disease, chickenpox, herpesvirus, molluscum contagiosum, warts, cold sores, shingles (herpes zoster), and others 2. Skin infections and infestations: ringworm (fungus), scabies (parasite), impetigo (bacteria)	• Skin may show similar findings with many different causes. Determining cause of rash requires a competent health professional evaluation that takes into account information other than just how rash looks.	• For outbreaks	Yes	**No, unless** • Rash with behavior change or fever • Has oozing/open wound • Has bruising not associated with injury • Has joint pain and rash • Unable to participate	• Able to participate in daily activities. • On medication at least 24 hours (if indicated). • Exclusion criteria are resolved.

Symptom	Common Causes	Complaints or What Might Be Seen	Notify Health Consultant	Notify Parent	Temporarily Exclude? (See also "When to Get Immediate Medical Help" on page 27).	If Excluded, Readmit When
Rash, continued	3. Severe bacterial infections: meningococcus, pneumococcus	1. Viral: Usually signs of general illness such as runny nose, cough, and fever (except for warts or molluscum). Each viral rash may have a distinctive appearance. 2. Skin infections and infestations: See "Itching." 3. Severe bacterial infections: Rare. These children have fever with rash and may be very ill.				
Sore Throat (pharyngitis)	1. Common cold viruses (upper respiratory infection) 2. Strep throat	1. Verbal children will complain of sore throat; younger children may be irritable with decreased appetite and increased drooling (refusal to swallow). May see symptoms associated with upper respiratory illness such as runny nose, cough, and congestion. 2. Strep infection usually does not result in cough or runny nose. Signs of the body's fight against infection include red tissue with white patches on sides of throat, at back of tongue (tonsil area), and at back wall of throat. Tonsils may be large, even touching each other. Swollen lymph nodes (sometimes incorrectly called "swollen glands") occur as body fights off the infection.		Yes	**No, unless** • Inability to swallow. • Excessive drooling with breathing difficulty. • Fever with behavior change. • The child meets other exclusion criteria (see "Conditions Requiring Temporary Exclusion" on page 28).	• Able to swallow. • Able to participate. • On medication at least 24 hours (if strep). • Exclusion criteria are resolved.

Symptom	Common Causes	Complaints or What Might Be Seen	Notify Health Consultant	Notify Parent	Temporarily Exclude? (See also "When to Get Immediate Medical Help" on page 27).	If Excluded, Readmit When
Stomachache	1. Viral gastroenteritis or strep throat 2. Problems with internal organs such as intestine	1. Vomiting and diarrhea and/or cramping are signs of a viral infection of stomach and/or intestine. Strep throat may cause stomachache with sore throat, headache, and possible fever. If cough or runny nose is present, strep is very unlikely. 2. Persistent severe pain in abdomen.		Yes	**No, unless** • Severe pain causing child to double over or scream • Abdominal pain after injury • Bloody/black stools • No urine output for 8 hours • Diarrhea • Vomiting • Yellow skin/eyes • Fever with behavior change • Looks or acts very ill	• Pain resolves. • Able to participate. • Exclusion criteria are resolved.
Swollen Glands (properly called swollen lymph nodes)	1. A body defense against viral or bacterial infection in the area where lymph nodes are located (ie, in the neck for upper respiratory infection, pharyngitis) 2. Bacterial infection of lymph nodes	1. Swelling at front and sides of neck; fever; runny nose, sore throat, or other symptoms of respiratory infection 2. Swollen lymph nodes in groin or under arms; boils or redness, pain, and warmth indicating infection in arm or leg on same side as swollen glands		Yes	**No, unless** • Difficulty breathing or swallowing • Red, tender, warm glands • Fever with behavior change	• Child is on antibiotics (if indicated). • Able to participate. • Exclusion criteria are resolved.
Vomiting	• Viral infection of the stomach or intestine (gastroenteritis) • Coughing strongly • Other viral illness with fever	Diarrhea, vomiting, and/or cramping for viral gastroenteritis	• For outbreak	Yes	**Yes, if** • Vomited more than 2 times in 24 hours • Vomiting and fever • Vomit that appears green/bloody • No urine output in 8 hours • Recent history of head injury • Looks or acts very ill	• Vomiting ends

CHAPTER 7

Quick Reference Sheets

The following section contains a series of quick reference sheets about some of the infections and infestations that commonly occur in children in group care settings. These are specific conditions or diseases that occur frequently, that sometimes cause concern for the public, or for which vaccines are given routinely. These conditions and diseases are arranged in alphabetic order according to what they are commonly called, not their scientific names (ie, chickenpox instead of varicella zoster).

Each sheet contains information about common signs and symptoms, incubation and contagious periods, spread, infection control, the role of the parent or caregiver/teacher, and exclusion and return-to-care criteria. Copy these quick reference sheets to facilitate communication among parents, caregivers/teachers, and pediatric health professionals. No permission is necessary to make single copies for noncommercial, educational purposes.

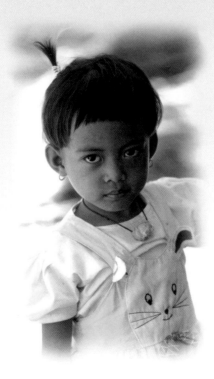

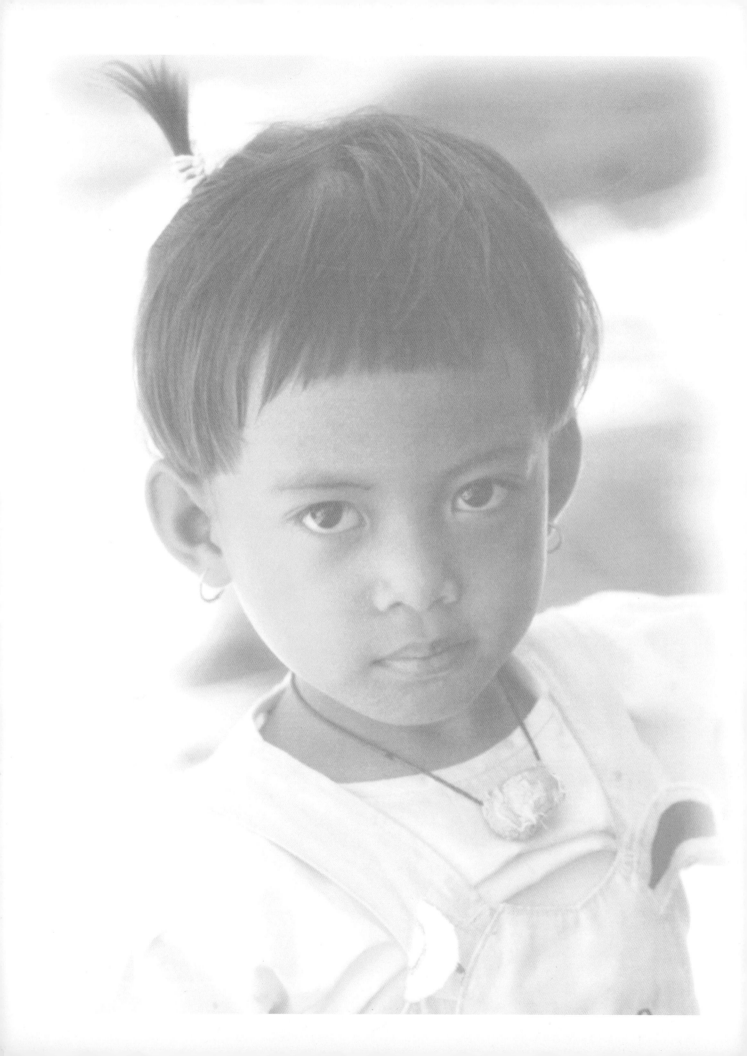

Bites (Human and Animal)

Human Bites

Biting is very common among young children, but usually does not cause serious injury. If the skin is broken, bacteria introduced into the wound can cause a tissue infection that needs treatment by a health professional. If blood is drawn into the mouth of the biter, or if the biter breaks the skin and has bleeding gums or mouth sores, blood-borne disease could be a concern. Hepatitis B virus, human immunodeficiency virus (HIV), and hepatitis C virus are examples of blood-borne pathogens. The risk of transmission of one of these viruses, however, is very low in child care and school settings. For HIV, no known transmission in a child care setting or school has occurred.

What are the roles of the caregiver/teacher and the family?

- Provide first aid by washing any broken skin and applying cold to any bruise.
- Notify the parent/guardian of a bite.
- Recommend a health professional visit if the skin is broken because preventive antibiotics may be indicated.
- Focus on the injured child, rather than on a child who is biting. Later, try to determine why the biting happened, to see if the situation can be prevented before biting occurs, and an alternative behavior could be suggested to the child who is biting (eg, using words or another acceptable behavior to express feelings).

Exclude from group setting?

No, unless the child is unable to participate and staff determine that they cannot care for the child without compromising their ability to care for the health and safety of the other children in the group.

Readmit to group setting?

When the child is able to participate and staff determine that they can care for the child without compromising their ability to care for the health and safety of the other children in the group.

Animal Bites

Reptiles should not be kept as pets for children and should not be allowed in any child care program or school. *Salmonella* inhabits the gastrointestinal tract and, thus, the environment of the reptiles. Therefore, contact with reptiles (eg, skin, environment) may cause *Salmonella* infection in children in schools and child care settings. Additionally, bites from reptiles may result in a *Salmonella* or other bacterial infection.

An animal bite that breaks or punctures the skin has a significant chance of producing a bacterial infection. Any wild animal or pet bite that breaks the skin should be evaluated by a health professional for the need for preventive antibiotics. Animal bites are common, and (uncommonly) bites of some animals (eg, stray dogs, raccoons, bats) may transmit rabies virus.

Rabies is a very serious viral infection that infects the nervous system. Rabies usually is transmitted by a variety of wild animals. However, the virus can be spread by unimmunized pets and, in rare cases, immunized pets that get infected. If a pet or wild animal bites someone and breaks the skin, the situation requires immediate attention. The person who was bitten may need to begin immediate treatment, and the animal should be observed by a veterinarian for signs of rabies. The risk is greatest when the animal is unimmunized and the bite was unprovoked. The virus spreads from the animal's saliva entering the bite site. Report all suspected exposure to rabies promptly to public health authorities and be sure health professionals are involved in deciding about appropriate treatment right away.

Signs or symptoms of rabies include anxiety, difficulty swallowing, seizures, and paralysis. Once signs or symptoms develop, rabies is nearly always a fatal disease.

How do you control it?

- By immunizing dogs and cats.
- By avoiding contact with wild or stray animals, particularly those acting peculiarly or aggressively. Children should not be allowed to touch dead animals.

➤ *continued*

Bites (Human and Animal), continued

What are the roles of the caregiver/teacher and the family?

- Provide first aid by washing any broken skin and applying cold to any bruise. Teach children to avoid contact with stray or dead animals.
- Make sure any animal in a child's environment is healthy and a suitable pet for children, fully immunized, and on a flea, tick, and worm-control program (when appropriate). A time-specified certificate from a veterinarian, indicating that the pet meets these conditions, should be on file.
- All contact between animals and children should be supervised by a caregiver/teacher.
- Contact a health professional if a child or adult is bitten
  - ~ By a pet or unknown or wild animal.
  - ~ There is redness, swelling, drainage, or pain.
  - ~ The skin is broken.
- If you can do so safely, capture or confine the animal for an evaluation.
- If there is a chance that a person has been exposed to rabies, medical attention is imperative.

Exclude from group setting?

No, unless the child is unable to participate and staff determine that they cannot care for the child without compromising their ability to care for the health and safety of the other children in the group.

Readmit to group setting?

When the child is able to participate and staff determine that they can care for the child without compromising their ability to care for the health and safety of the other children in the group.

American Academy of Pediatrics

DEDICATED TO THE HEALTH OF ALL CHILDREN™

The American Academy of Pediatrics is an organization of 60,000 primary care pediatricians, pediatric medical subspecialists, and pediatric surgical specialists dedicated to the health, safety, and well-being of infants, children, adolescents, and young adults.

American Academy of Pediatrics
PO Box 747
Elk Grove Village, IL 60009-0747
Web site—http://www.aap.org

Campylobacter

What is *Campylobacter?*

A type of bacteria that can cause diarrheal infection

What are the signs or symptoms?

- Bloody diarrhea
- Fever
- Vomiting
- Abdominal cramping
- Malaise

What are the incubation and contagious periods?

- Incubation period: 1 to 7 days, but can be longer.
- Contagious period: Excretion of *Campylobacter* is shortened by treatment. Without treatment, excretion of bacteria can continue for 2 to 3 weeks, and relapse of symptoms may occur.

How is it spread?

- Contact with stool from infected birds, farm animals (eg, chickens and turkeys), or pets (eg, dogs, cats, hamsters, birds—especially young animals)
- Contaminated water
- Unpasteurized milk
- Contaminated food (eg, raw poultry)
- Person-to-person via the fecal-oral route occurs occasionally, particularly from very young children (most likely during diarrhea phase)

How do you control it?

- Proper hand washing, particularly after contact with raw poultry or dog or cat feces
- Exclusion for specific types of symptoms (see "Exclude from group setting?")
- Antibiotics

What are the roles of the caregiver/teacher and the family?

- Report the infection to staff designated by the child care program or school for decision making and action related to care of ill children. That person, in turn, alerts possibly exposed family members and staff to watch for symptoms.
- Report the infection to the health department, as the health professional who makes the diagnosis may not report that the child who has the infection is a participant in a child care program or school, and this could lead to loss of precious time for controlling the spread of the disease.
- Conduct ongoing education for staff addressing transmission, control, and prevention of diarrheal diseases.
- Use good hand washing and food sanitation techniques, especially after handling raw poultry, dogs, and cats.
- Avoid milk that is not pasteurized and water that is not chlorinated.

Exclude from group setting?

Yes, if

- Any child or caregiver/teacher has bloody diarrhea or any child with diarrhea cannot contain the diarrhea completely with the use of the toilet, unless children with symptoms can be cared for in a completely separate area until diarrhea is resolved (all children in diapers with diarrhea must be excluded).
- The child is unable to participate and staff determine that they cannot care for the child without compromising their ability to care for the health and safety of the other children in the group.
- The child meets other exclusion criteria, such as fever with behavior change (see "Conditions Requiring Temporary Exclusion" on page 28).

Readmit to group setting?

- When diarrhea has resolved or reverted to a new stool pattern for more than a week (Note: It is not necessary to demonstrate negative stool cultures as long as the child's symptoms have resolved.)
- When the child is able to participate and staff determine that they can care for the child without compromising their ability to care for the health and safety of the other children in the group

Comments

- Antibiotics will shorten illness time and clear bacteria from stool faster.
- Outbreaks are uncommon in group care settings.

American Academy of Pediatrics

DEDICATED TO THE HEALTH OF ALL CHILDREN™

The American Academy of Pediatrics is an organization of 60,000 primary care pediatricians, pediatric medical subspecialists, and pediatric surgical specialists dedicated to the health, safety, and well-being of infants, children, adolescents, and young adults.

American Academy of Pediatrics
PO Box 747
Elk Grove Village, IL 60009-0747
Web site—http://www.aap.org

Chickenpox (Varicella-Zoster Infections)

What is chickenpox?

A respiratory illness caused by the varicella-zoster virus

What are the signs or symptoms?

- Rash (ie, small, red bumps blistering over 3–4 days, then forming scabs).
- Blister crops will come out over several days, so the person who has chickenpox for more than a day or so will have some red bumps, blisters, and scabbed-over blisters all at the same time.
- Rash is more noticeable on the trunk than exposed parts of the body.
- Rash may appear inside mouth, ears, genital areas, and scalp.
- Fever, runny nose, cough.

What are the incubation and contagious periods?

- Incubation period: Usually 14 to 16 days, occasionally as short as 10 days and as long as 21 days after contact.
- Contagious period: The most contagious period is from 1 to 2 days before the rash appears until right after it appears. An infected person no longer spreads the virus when all the blisters have scabs and no new blisters are forming.

How is it spread?

- Chickenpox is highly contagious. Even brief exposure or shared airflow poses a high risk of infection for people who have not had the disease before or have not been protected by the chickenpox vaccine.
- Primarily from direct contact with mucus from the eyes, nose, or mouth and from fluid inside the blisters of an infected person.
- Airborne via mouth or nose droplets from coughing or sneezing.
- Can be spread by someone with uncovered shingles lesions, as the virus that causes shingles is reactivated chickenpox virus in someone who previously had chickenpox.

How do you control it?

- Vaccinate all children 12 months of age or older.
- Vaccinate young adults and other adults who are susceptible.
- Exclude infected children and caregivers/teachers until rash is crusted over.

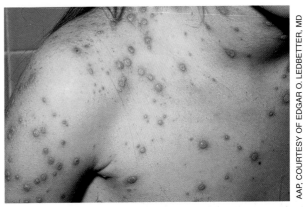

Child with chickenpox rash

AAP, COURTESY OF EDGAR O. LEDBETTER, MD

- Practice good hand washing and surface sanitation.
- Ventilate room air with fresh outdoor air.
  - ~ Children with chickenpox who are mildly ill and able to come to a program that cares for children who are ill require a room with separate ventilation with exhaust to and air exchange with the outside.
- Exclusion for a chickenpox rash is necessary even if the child has received varicella vaccine, unless the child can have a viral culture performed that determines the virus is from the vaccine and not wild chickenpox virus and the lesions can be covered.

What are the roles of the caregiver/teacher and the family?

- Report the infection to staff designated by the child care program or school for decision making and action related to care of ill children. That person, in turn, alerts possibly exposed family members and staff to watch for symptoms.
- Report the infection to the health department, as the health professional who makes the diagnosis may not report that the child who has the infection is a participant in a child care program or school, and this could lead to precious time for controlling the spread of the disease being lost.
- Specifically notify all adults who have not had chickenpox or the chickenpox vaccine and who may have been exposed (eg, families, staff, volunteers—especially those who are or might be pregnant or have an immune system disease). Suggest that they check with their health professionals about what to do.
- Wash hands carefully at routine times (see "Hand Washing Steps" on page 17) and after any contact with soiled articles or blisters.

➤ continued

Chickenpox (Varicella-Zoster Infections), continued

- Do not give aspirin to children who are ill, as it may increase their risk of contracting Reye syndrome, a serious complication associated with the use of aspirin in someone infected with chickenpox and other viral illnesses (eg, influenza).
- Pregnant women should be referred to their health professional within 24 hours after exposure to chickenpox. Pregnant women who previously have had chickenpox should not have a pregnancy-related problem if exposed to chickenpox. However, pregnant women should be encouraged to confirm their protection with their own health professionals.

Exclude from group setting?

Yes. Chickenpox is a highly communicable illness for which routine exclusion of infected children is warranted.

Readmit to group setting?

- When all blisters have scabs (usually 6 days after start of rash).
- When the child is able to participate and staff determine that they can care for the child without compromising their ability to care for the health and safety of the other children in the group

Comments

- Virus can stay for a lifetime in an inactive form in the body's nerve cells.
- Shingles (herpes zoster) is the condition that occurs if the inactive virus becomes active (see "Shingles (Herpes Zoster)" on page 119).
- Rash from varicella vaccination can occur in 3% to 5% of children 5 to 26 days after vaccination. This condition is mild and usually causes only a few red bumps at or near the injection site. Bumps near the injection site may be covered with a nonporous bandage and clothing and the child may continue to participate. Occasionally, the rash after varicella vaccination may be more widespread. Although this condition is not contagious to others through the respiratory route, it is difficult to tell whether a widespread chickenpox rash is caused by the vaccine or a natural infection. Therefore, any child with a widespread varicella rash must be excluded until all blisters have scabs.
- Rarely, children get chickenpox a second time. These cases usually are very mild with less fever and fewer bumps and blisters than the first time.
- It is possible for children to get chickenpox despite being vaccinated. The vaccine is only about 70% to 85% effective against mild disease (although 95% effective at preventing severe chickenpox). Chickenpox in previously immunized children usually is mild with less fever and fewer bumps and blisters than in unimmunized children.

American Academy of Pediatrics

DEDICATED TO THE HEALTH OF ALL CHILDREN™

The American Academy of Pediatrics is an organization of 60,000 primary care pediatricians, pediatric medical subspecialists, and pediatric surgical specialists dedicated to the health, safety, and well-being of infants, children, adolescents, and young adults.

American Academy of Pediatrics
PO Box 747
Elk Grove Village, IL 60009-0747
Web site—http://www.aap.org

Common Skin Warts (Human Papillomavirus)

What are common skin warts?

Skin infections caused by the human papillomavirus

What are the signs or symptoms?

- Dome-shaped growth inside the skin that may become a raised area with small bumps within it.
- Usually painless, but may be painful when they occur on the feet.
- Often found on the hands and around or under fingernails.
- Black dots may appear in the warts.

What are the incubation and contagious periods?

- Incubation period: Unknown, but estimated to range from 3 months to several years.
- Contagious period: Unknown, but probably as long as the wart is present.

How are they spread?

Person-to-person through close contact

How do you control them?

- Wash hands after touching the warts.
- Do not share towels used by an infected child or caregiver/teacher.
- Scratching the warts may cause further bacterial infection or spread of virus to other sites.
- The body may make antibodies to the virus that causes the wart so that the wart spontaneously resolves.
- Alternatively, treatments may be used. Tissue-destructive treatments such as medicated tape and liquid nitrogen may activate the body's immune response to the virus that causes the wart and hasten the resolution of the warts. However, treated warts may return and often require re-treatment.
- Although warts are a viral infection, they are very mildly contagious and most often are spread to other areas of the affected child's body, rather than to other children. Warts do not need to be covered like shingles or other oozing sores. Treatment is a personal choice and not an infection control issue for a group care setting.

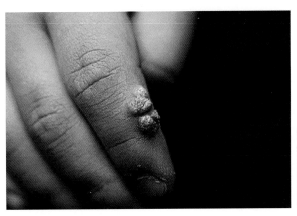

Child with wart on finger

GARY WILLIAMS, MD

What are the roles of the caregiver/teacher and the family?

- Practice careful and frequent hand washing after contact with the child's warts.
- Do not let children pick at their warts because this may cause an opening in the skin promoting bacterial infection.

Exclude from group setting?

No.

Comments

- Many people have warts at some time in their lives.
- Immunocompromised children, including those with HIV infection, may have more severe and widespread lesions.

American Academy
of Pediatrics

DEDICATED TO THE HEALTH OF ALL CHILDREN™

The American Academy of Pediatrics is an organization of 60,000 primary care pediatricians, pediatric medical subspecialists, and pediatric surgical specialists dedicated to the health, safety, and well-being of infants, children, adolescents, and young adults.

American Academy of Pediatrics
PO Box 747
Elk Grove Village, IL 60009-0747
Web site—http://www.aap.org

Cytomegalovirus (CMV)

What is cytomegalovirus?

A viral infection common in children (Up to 70% of normal children 1 to 3 years of age in group care settings excrete CMV.)

What are the signs or symptoms?

- Often mild to no symptoms in children.
- Adults may have a mononucleosis type of illness with fever; sometimes the liver or spleen may become enlarged.

What are the incubation and contagious periods?

Unknown for person-to-person transmission

How is it spread?

- Direct person-to-person contact with infected secretions and urine
- Mother to infant before, during, and after birth
- Blood transfusions from an infected person

How do you control it?

Attention to proper hand washing, especially by women of childbearing age working with young children

What are the roles of the caregiver/teacher and the family?

- Careful hand washing for staff and family members.
- Review of standard precautions, particularly hand hygiene, especially for women working with children younger than 3 years.
- Women of childbearing age who have any contact with children in group care settings should discuss the risk of CMV with their health professionals.

Exclude from group setting?

No, unless

- The child is unable to participate and staff determine that they cannot care for the child without compromising their ability to care for the health and safety of the other children in the group.
- The child meets other exclusion criteria, such as fever with behavior change (see "Conditions Requiring Temporary Exclusion" on page 28).

Readmit to group setting?

When exclusion criteria are resolved, the child is able to participate, and staff determine that they can care for the child without compromising their ability to care for the health and safety of the other children in the group.

Comments

- Individuals remain infectious as long as the virus is in body secretions, which can be months or years. Because this virus is so common in child care settings, exclusion to reduce disease transmission has no benefit.
- A blood test for CMV antibodies will show whether a woman is already immune or susceptible to CMV. Testing children for excretion of the virus or performing CMV antibody tests on children because they are in a group care setting is inappropriate.

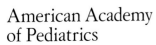

American Academy of Pediatrics

DEDICATED TO THE HEALTH OF ALL CHILDREN™

The American Academy of Pediatrics is an organization of 60,000 primary care pediatricians, pediatric medical subspecialists, and pediatric surgical specialists dedicated to the health, safety, and well-being of infants, children, adolescents, and young adults.

American Academy of Pediatrics
PO Box 747
Elk Grove Village, IL 60009-0747
Web site—http://www.aap.org

Copyright © 2005 American Academy of Pediatrics

Diaper Rash/Thrush (Candidiasis)

What is diaper rash?

A shiny red rash, pinker than usual skin, or red bumps in the diaper area that may be caused by *Candida*. There are other causes of diaper rash that produce a similar skin appearance.

What is thrush?

A yeast infection predominately produced by the *Candida albicans* organism causing mouth infections in young infants

What are the signs or symptoms?

- Of *Candida* diaper rash
  ~ Redness in the diaper area.
  ~ Worse in the creases.
  ~ Redness often bordered by red pimples.
  ~ Rash may have a shiny appearance.
  ~ Sores or cracking or oozing skin present in severe cases.
- Of thrush
  ~ White patches on the inside of cheeks and on gums and tongue.
  ~ Usually causes no other signs or symptoms.

What are the incubation and contagious periods?

- Incubation period: Unknown.
- Contagious period: The yeast that causes thrush and infects the diaper area is widespread in the environment, normally lives on the skin, and is found in the mouth and stool. Mild infection of the lining of the mouth is common in healthy infants. Thrush and *Candida* diaper rash may occur with antibiotic use. Repetitive or severe thrush and *Candida* diaper rash could signal immune problems.

How are they spread?

- *Candida albicans* is present in the intestinal tract and mucous membranes of healthy people.
- A warm environment (eg, mouth, diaper area) fosters growth and spread.

- Person-to-person transmission may occur from a woman to her infant when the mother has a yeast infection in her vagina and in breastfeeding mothers whose babies with thrush infect the mothers' nipples.

How do you control them?

- Hand washing.
- Treatment of individuals who have an infection so that the quantity of the fungus in any area is reduced to levels that the body can control.
- Wash and sanitize toys, bottle and pacifier nipples, and utensils that have been mouthed before allowing sharing with another child.

What are the roles of the caregiver/teacher and the family?

- Report the infection to staff designated by the child care program or school for decision making and action related to care of ill children. That person, in turn, alerts possibly exposed family members and staff to watch for symptoms.
- Administer prescribed medication as instructed by the child's health professional.

Exclude from group setting?

No.

American Academy of Pediatrics

DEDICATED TO THE HEALTH OF ALL CHILDREN™

The American Academy of Pediatrics is an organization of 60,000 primary care pediatricians, pediatric medical subspecialists, and pediatric surgical specialists dedicated to the health, safety, and well-being of infants, children, adolescents, and young adults.

American Academy of Pediatrics
PO Box 747
Elk Grove Village, IL 60009-0747
Web site—http://www.aap.org

Diarrhea

What is diarrhea?

An illness that is defined by more watery stools, less-formed stools, and increased frequency of stools. Diarrhea can be caused by changes in diet, such as eating more than the usual amounts of certain foods, and the use of some medications. Infectious causes include viruses, bacteria, and parasites.

- Viruses: rotaviruses, enteric adenoviruses, astroviruses, caliciviruses, hepatitis A, enteroviruses
- Bacteria: *Shigella, Salmonella, Campylobacter, Escherichia coli* O157:H7, *Clostridium difficile*
- Parasites: *Giardia lamblia, Cryptosporidium parvum*

What are the signs or symptoms?

- Frequent loose or watery stools.
- Abdominal cramps and tenderness.
- Fever.
- Generally not feeling well.
- Blood in stool.
- Individuals can be infected and infectious with minimal signs or symptoms.

What are the incubation and contagious periods?

See specific disease sheets.

How is it spread?

- Fecal-oral route (fecally contaminated food, hands, or surfaces touched by objects or hands put into the mouth)
- Water contaminated by human or animal feces (eg, swimming pools)
- Trips to sites with animals (eg, farms, pet stores, petting zoos)

What are some types of diarrhea?

- Viruses cause the majority of diarrheal illness in group care settings. The most common virus associated with diarrhea in the winter months is rotavirus, which causes watery diarrhea. Enteroviruses are more common in the summer. Other viral infections may include diarrhea as one symptom (see specific disease sheets for more information).
- Diarrheal infections from bacteria are uncommon, but may cause bloody diarrhea. A health professional always should evaluate anyone with bloody diarrhea. The evaluation should include one or more tests or stool cultures to identify the type of bacteria involved.

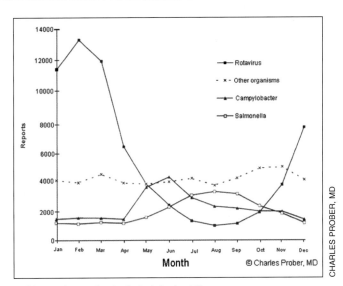

CHARLES PROBER, MD

Incidences by month of selected diarrheal illnesses

How do you control it?

- Careful and frequent hand washing is essential, especially after toilet use or handling soiled diapers and before anything to do with food preparation or eating.
- Proper cooking and storage of food.
- Exclusion of infected staff who handle food.
- Exclusion of children with signs or symptoms who cannot use the toilet (all infants and children in diapers or who have toileting "accidents").
  ~ Families should not bring to the facility and should remove from the facility any child with diarrhea who cannot use a toilet for all bowel movements while in the group care setting. Pending arrival of a parent/guardian, the child should not have contact with other children or be placed in areas used by caregivers/teachers who have contact with other children in the facility. This can be accomplished by moving the ill child to a separate area of the facility or, if that is not possible, to a separate area of the room where the child usually stays. The area should be supervised by a caregiver/teacher known to the child, and the toys, equipment, and surfaces must not be used by any other child or caregiver/teacher until after the ill child leaves and all surfaces have been sanitized.
  ~ When moving a child to a separate area of the facility would cause problems with supervision of the other children, the ill child should be kept as comfortable as possible in the child's usual area, with minimal contact between ill and well children, until the family member arrives to remove the child.

➤ *continued*

Diarrhea, continued

What are the roles of the caregiver/teacher and the family?

- Report the infection to staff designated by the child care program or school for decision making and action related to care of ill children. That person, in turn, alerts possibly exposed family members and staff to watch for symptoms.
- Ensure that staff follow strict and frequent hand washing, diapering, toileting, food handling and cleaning, and sanitation procedures.
- Stop food handling or feeding of others by individuals with diarrhea.
- Report outbreaks of diarrhea (more than 2 children in the group) to the health department.

Exclude from group setting?

Yes, if

- Child has
  - ~ Diarrhea not contained in the toilet (All infants and children in diapers with diarrhea must be excluded.)
  - ~ Blood or mucus in stool
  - ~ Abnormal color of stool for that child (eg, all black or very pale)
  - ~ No urine output in 8 hours
  - ~ Fever and behavior change
  - ~ Jaundice (ie, yellow skin or eyes)
  - ~ The appearance of being ill
- The child is unable to participate and staff determine that they cannot care for the child without compromising their ability to care for the health and safety of the other children in the group.

Readmit to group setting?

- A health professional must clear the child for readmission for all cases of bloody diarrhea and diarrhea caused by *Shigella, Salmonella, E coli* O157:H7, or *G lamblia*. Children with *Shigella* and *E coli* O157:H7 are excluded until diarrhea resolves and test results from 2 stool cultures at least 24 hours apart are negative for these bacteria. Children with *Salmonella typhi* are excluded until 3 stool cultures taken at least 24 hours apart are negative for these bacteria.
- Stool is contained in toilet (for toilet-trained children).
- Even if stools stay loose, may readmit when the child seems well and the stool consistency has not changed for a week.
- When the child is able to participate and staff determine that they can care for the child without compromising their ability to care for the health and safety of the other children in the group.

American Academy
of Pediatrics

DEDICATED TO THE HEALTH OF ALL CHILDREN™

The American Academy of Pediatrics is an organization of 60,000 primary care pediatricians, pediatric medical subspecialists, and pediatric surgical specialists dedicated to the health, safety, and well-being of infants, children, adolescents, and young adults.

American Academy of Pediatrics
PO Box 747
Elk Grove Village, IL 60009-0747
Web site—http://www.aap.org

Ear Infection

What is an ear infection?

Although ear infections can occur in the ear canal and in the inner ear, most ear infections of young children occur in the middle ear. The middle ear is the space behind the eardrum where tiny bones attached to the eardrum transmit sound across the air space of the middle ear to the inner ear. An infection of the middle ear is called *otitis media.*

An infection of the ear canal can occur when bacteria infect the skin that lines the canal. This most commonly occurs from swimming. Moisture from the pool, lake, or stream promotes bacterial growth and infection of the skin of the ear canal, producing painful swelling and inflammation. Pus may collect in the ear canal. This type of ear infection is called swimmer's ear, or *otitis externa.*

An ear infection of the middle ear most often occurs when mucus from a cold, allergy, or some other irritation of the respiratory tract accumulates in the middle ear space. This occurs more easily in small children because the tube that normally drains the middle ear is small, more horizontal than later in life, and easily blocked. The drainage tube is called the eustachian tube.

Ear infections can be very painful, but most resolve by themselves in a day or two. Viruses cause most middle ear infections. Inexperience of the immune system, small structures, and frequent colds that keep putting fluid into the middle ear increase the risk for ear infection.

Although the majority of all children get ear infections when they are young, children who are in group care are more likely to get ear infections. Also, children who lie on their backs to drink from a bottle are more prone to ear infections. The increased risk from feeding position may be due to milk getting into the opening of the eustachian tube in the back of the throat, causing irritation and blockage.

What are the signs or symptoms?

- Pain inside the ear or when moving the ear lobe
- Fussing and crying while sucking
- May have fever
- Ear drainage

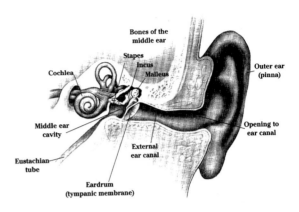

Cross Section of the Ear

What are the incubation and contagious periods?

- Incubation period: Related to the type of virus or bacteria that is causing the fluid buildup in the middle ear. For ear canal infections, signs or symptoms usually appear within a day or so after swimming.
- Contagious period: Ear infections are not contagious. The virus or bacteria that led to the ear infection may be contagious, but by the time a middle ear infection has developed the infection that caused the ear infection is usually not very contagious.

How is it spread?

Ear infections are not contagious. They are a complication of a respiratory infection or a bacterial infection of the skin in the ear canal.

How do you control it?

- For a middle ear infection
  - ~ Keep the child with a respiratory infection well-hydrated—offering water to drink frequently.
  - ~ Keep room air from being too dry, which tends to dry out the secretions and make them thicker and harder to drain. Ventilate the facility with fresh outdoor air and maintain temperature and humidity conditions as described in *Caring for Our Children,* Standard 5.028.
    - ❖ Winter months: 65°F to 75°F with 30% to 50% relative humidity
    - ❖ Summer months: 68°F to 82°F with 30% to 50% relative humidity
    - ❖ Air exchange: Minimum of 15 cubic feet per minute per person of outdoor air

➤ *continued*

Ear Infection, continued

~ Get treatment instructions from a health professional. Sometimes eardrops that numb the eardrum or an oral pain reducing medication (ie, acetaminophen or ibuprofen) are all that is needed. Sometimes the health professional will prescribe antibiotics.
- For an ear canal infection
  ~ Prevent infection by rinsing out ear canals with clean water after swimming. Sometimes health professionals will recommend a special ear wash after swimming if the child has a lot of trouble with ear canal infections.
  ~ Dry the ears by allowing the water to drain out onto a towel.
  ~ Get treatment instructions from a health professional.
- For a child with ear drainage
  ~ Have child evaluated by a health professional

What are the roles of the caregiver/teacher and the family?

Observe the child's signs or symptoms and arrange for family members to contact the child's health professional for management instructions.

Exclude from group setting?

No, unless

- The child is unable to participate and staff determine that they cannot care for the child without compromising their ability to care for the health and safety of the other children in the group.
- The child meets other exclusion criteria, such as fever with behavior change (see "Conditions Requiring Temporary Exclusion" on page 28).

Readmit to group setting?

When exclusion criteria are resolved, the child is able to participate, and staff determine that they can care for the child without compromising their ability to care for the health and safety of the other children in the group

Comments

Ear infections can be very trying for children, families, and caregiver/teachers. Sometimes, with repeated ear infections, hearing may be temporarily impaired. Some children have trouble with blockage of their eustachian tubes for a long time, so the fluid stays trapped in the middle ear. In these cases, health professionals may place a drainage tube through their eardrum. The tube allows fluid to drain from the middle ear into the ear canal and air from the ear canal to enter the middle ear space until all the structures are fully healed.

American Academy of Pediatrics

DEDICATED TO THE HEALTH OF ALL CHILDREN™

The American Academy of Pediatrics is an organization of 60,000 primary care pediatricians, pediatric medical subspecialists, and pediatric surgical specialists dedicated to the health, safety, and well-being of infants, children, adolescents, and young adults.

American Academy of Pediatrics
PO Box 747
Elk Grove Village, IL 60009-0747
Web site—http://www.aap.org

Escherichia coli Diarrhea

What is *Escherichia coli* diarrhea?

Although many types of *E coli* bacteria live normally in the intestinal tract, at least 5 types are known to cause diarrhea. Two types, enteropathogenic *E coli* and *E coli* O157:H7 have caused numerous outbreaks in group care settings. Infections with *E coli* O157:H7 may be associated with other severe problems such as bleeding from irritation of the bowel, kidney damage, and blood cell damage, also known as hemolytic uremic syndrome.

What are the signs or symptoms?

- Loose stools, which may be watery and bloody
- Abdominal pain
- May have fever

What are the incubation and contagious periods?

- Incubation period: 10 hours to 6 days; *E coli* O157:H7 averages 3 to 5 days, but ranges from 1 to 8 days.
- Contagious period: Until diarrhea resolves and test results from 2 consecutive stool cultures are negative for the *E coli* bacteria that caused the problem.

How is it spread?

- Direct contact with infected and symptomatic people
- Food or water contaminated with human and animal feces (eg, cattle, sheep, deer, undercooked ground beef, unpasteurized milk, or other products contaminated with cattle feces such as contaminated apple cider, raw vegetables, salami, yogurt, and untreated drinking water in recreation areas)
- Can be brought back by those who have visited developing countries

How do you control it?

- Cook all ground beef thoroughly so there is no pink meat.
- Use only pasteurized milk and apple juice products.
- Immediately involve pubic health authorities when a case of diarrhea occurs that is attributable to *E coli* O157:H7.

- Exclude ill children until diarrhea resolves and test results from 2 consecutive stool cultures are negative for the bacteria.
- Close the facility to any new admissions.
- Prevent enrolled children from being transferred for care to other groups or facilities where they may expose other susceptible children.
- Strict attention to hand washing.
- Sanitation or disposal of contaminated items.

What are the roles of the caregiver/teacher and the family?

- Report the infection to staff designated by the child care program or school for decision making and action related to care of ill children. That person, in turn, alerts possibly exposed family members and staff to watch for symptoms.
- Report the infection to the health department, as the health professional who makes the diagnosis may not report that the child who has the infection is a participant in a child care program or school, and this could lead to precious time for controlling the spread of the disease being lost.
- Institute control measures.

Exclude from group setting?
Yes.

Readmit to group setting?

- When diarrhea resolves and test results from 2 consecutive stool cultures taken 24 hours apart are negative for the bacteria that caused the illness
- When the child is able to participate and staff determine that they can care for the child without compromising their ability to care for the health and safety of the other children in the group

Comments

- Outbreaks of *E coli* diarrhea have been associated with the death of young children. Management requires informing parents/guardians carefully about the problem, identifying the source of contamination, and containing the spread of disease with the recommended control measures.

➤ *continued*

Escherichia coli Diarrhea, continued

- Many group care settings include visits to petting zoos or by animals into the classroom as a routine activity. The risk of exposure of young children to animal feces in such activities is very high. The feces are picked up on all body parts of the animal as it lies in bedding materials or brushes against other animals. Many petting zoos provide hand washing facilities adjacent to the animal contact areas now. Nevertheless, even with great vigilance on the part of caregivers/teachers, young children are very likely to touch an animal or have their skin and clothing touched by an animal and then put their contaminated hands or something touched with their contaminated hands into their mouths—even when hand washing sinks are available. Even with an adult-child ratio of 1:1, safely managing this contamination when dealing with infants, toddlers, and young preschool-aged children is extremely difficult. The significant risks of such animal contact should be weighed against the benefits.

American Academy
of Pediatrics

DEDICATED TO THE HEALTH OF ALL CHILDREN™

The American Academy of Pediatrics is an organization of 60,000 primary care pediatricians, pediatric medical subspecialists, and pediatric surgical specialists dedicated to the health, safety, and well-being of infants, children, adolescents, and young adults.

American Academy of Pediatrics
PO Box 747
Elk Grove Village, IL 60009-0747
Web site—http://www.aap.org

Fifth Disease (Human Parvovirus B19)

What is fifth disease?

Common viral infection with rash occurring 1 to 3 weeks after infection

What are the signs or symptoms?

- Fever.
- Muscle aches.
- May cause joint pain (uncommon in children, but more common in adults).
- Headache.
- Red "slapped-cheek" rash 1 to 3 weeks after these signs or symptoms. This characteristic rash is followed shortly by a lace-like appearing rash proceeding from trunk to arms, buttocks, and thighs.
  ~ Rash may disappear and reappear after exposure to heat for weeks; once rash appears, the child no longer feels ill.
- Individuals can be infected and infectious without ever having any signs or symptoms.
- Disease can be severe in people with sickle cell disease or certain blood disorders as well as those with compromised immune systems.

What are the incubation and contagious periods?

- Incubation period: 4 to 14 days, but can be as long as 21 days
- Contagious period: Until the rash appears (except in rare cases of infection in patients with certain blood disorders or compromised immune functions)

How is it spread?

- Direct contact with respiratory secretions (outbreaks occur in late winter and early spring.)
- Exposure to blood or blood products
- Exposure of a fetus in the uterus of a mother who becomes infected during pregnancy

How do you control it?

- Hand washing
- Sanitation of contaminated items
- Disposal of tissues containing nose and throat secretions

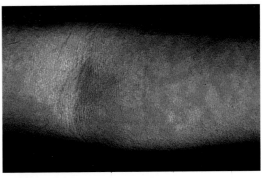

Child's arm with lace-like appearing rash

AAP, COURTESY OF EDGAR O. LEDBETTER, MD

What are the roles of the caregiver/teacher and the family?

- Report the infection to staff designated by the child care program or school for decision making and action related to care of ill children. That person, in turn, alerts possibly exposed family members and staff to watch for symptoms.
- Susceptible pregnant caregivers/teachers and pregnant mothers of children in child care and school settings should carefully wash their hands to reduce their risk of this infection and infection from other viruses that could harm a fetus.
- Teach children and caregivers/teachers to cover their noses and mouths when sneezing or coughing with a disposable facial tissue, if possible, or a shoulder if no facial tissue is available in time ("give your cough or sneeze a cold shoulder"). Teach everyone to remove any soil, change or cover contaminated clothing, and wash hands right after using facial tissues or having contact with mucus to prevent the spread of disease by contaminated hands.
- Dispose of facial tissues that contain nasal secretions after each use.

Exclude from group setting?

No, unless

- The child has sickle cell disease or a compromised immune system. Children with these conditions may shed large amounts of virus and may appear ill.
- The child is unable to participate and staff determine that they cannot care for the child without compromising their ability to care for the health and safety of the other children in the group.

➤ continued

Fifth Disease (Human Parvovirus B19), continued

- The child meets other exclusion criteria, such as fever with behavior change (see "Conditions Requiring Temporary Exclusion" on page 28).

Readmit to group setting?

When exclusion criteria are resolved, the child is able to participate, and staff determine that they can care for the child without compromising their ability to care for the health and safety of the other children in the group

Comments

Pregnant family members and caregivers/teachers who expect to have contact with children in group care settings should consult with their health professionals about their immune status and risk of infection. Women who are or may become pregnant and who work with children in group care settings can have a blood test to see if they are already immune to this virus. A positive test result may alleviate concern about the risk to their fetuses.

American Academy of Pediatrics

DEDICATED TO THE HEALTH OF ALL CHILDREN™

The American Academy of Pediatrics is an organization of 60,000 primary care pediatricians, pediatric medical subspecialists, and pediatric surgical specialists dedicated to the health, safety, and well-being of infants, children, adolescents, and young adults.

American Academy of Pediatrics
PO Box 747
Elk Grove Village, IL 60009-0747
Web site—http://www.aap.org

Giardiasis

What is Giardiasis?

An intestinal infection caused by a parasite *(Giardia lamblia)*

What are the signs or symptoms?

- Acute watery diarrhea.
- Excessive gas (flatulence, passing gas from the bowel).
- Distended and painful abdomen.
- Decreased appetite.
- Weight loss.
- Individuals can be infected and infectious without signs or symptoms.

What are the incubation and contagious periods?

- Incubation period: 1–4 weeks
- Contagious period: Highly variable, but can be months

How is it spread?

- Fecal-oral route
- Ingestion of contaminated water or food

How do you control it?

- Practice careful and frequent hand washing (see "Hand Washing Steps" on page 17).
- Identify and treat family members, staff, and children who have symptoms.
- Exclude people with diarrhea until they are symptom free.
- Note: Treatment and exclusion of carriers is not effective for outbreak control.

What are the roles of the caregiver/teacher and the family?

- Report the infection to staff designated by the child care program or school for decision making and action related to care of ill children. That person, in turn, alerts possibly exposed family members and staff to watch for symptoms.
- Report the infection to the health department, as the health professional who makes the diagnosis may not report that the child who has the infection is a participant in a child care program or school, and this could lead to precious time for controlling the spread of the disease being lost.
- Administer medication as prescribed.
- Emphasize sanitation and personal hygiene in the group care setting.
- Ensure that caregivers/teachers and children wash hands after toilet use or handling soiled diapers.
- Ensure that caregivers/teachers who care for diapered children do not prepare food for children outside their own group; try to arrange their duties with coworkers so that they do not participate in diaper changing until after they have completed their food preparation activities.

Exclude from group setting?

Yes, if

- Diarrhea is present.
- Note: For caregivers/teachers and children without symptoms (ie, recently recovered or exposed), testing stool cultures, treatment, and exclusion are not necessary.
- The child is unable to participate and staff determine that they cannot care for the child without compromising their ability to care for the health and safety of the other children in the group.

Readmit to group setting?

- Once diarrhea has resolved
- When the child is able to participate and staff determine that they can care for the child without compromising their ability to care for the health and safety of the other children in the group

Comments

- *Giardia* organisms are very common in the stools of young children in child care programs and schools.
- Outbreaks in group care settings may occur.

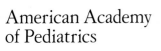

American Academy of Pediatrics

DEDICATED TO THE HEALTH OF ALL CHILDREN™

The American Academy of Pediatrics is an organization of 60,000 primary care pediatricians, pediatric medical subspecialists, and pediatric surgical specialists dedicated to the health, safety, and well-being of infants, children, adolescents, and young adults.

American Academy of Pediatrics
PO Box 747
Elk Grove Village, IL 60009-0747
Web site—http://www.aap.org

Haemophilus influenzae Type b (Hib)

What is *Haemophilus influenzae* type b?

- A bacteria that can infect ears, eyes, sinuses, epiglottis (ie, the flap that covers the windpipe), skin, lungs, blood, joints, throat, and coverings of the brain
- Not to be confused with "the flu"
- An infection that is generally prevented by routine childhood immunizations

What are the signs or symptoms?

Depends on the site of infection. May include
- Fever
- Vomiting
- Irritability
- Stiff neck
- Rapid onset of difficult breathing
- Cough
- Warm, red, swollen joints
- Swelling and discoloration of the skin, particularly of the cheek and around the eye

What are the incubation and contagious periods?

- Incubation period: Unknown
- Contagious period: Until antibiotic treatment has begun

How is it spread?

- Respiratory route
- Direct contact

How do you control it?

- Hib infection is a vaccine-preventable disease. Children should receive vaccine according to the most recent immunization recommendations.
- Giving a specific type of antibiotic to prevent the disease in exposed individuals should be considered. Such an approach would be worthwhile to prevent further spread of the disease.

- Report the infection to the health department, as the health professional who makes the diagnosis may not report that the child who has the infection is a participant in a child care program or school, and this could lead to precious time for controlling the spread of the disease being lost.

What are the roles of the caregiver/teacher and the family?

- Report the infection to staff designated by the child care program or school for decision making and action related to care of ill children. That person, in turn, alerts possibly exposed family members and staff to watch for symptoms.
- Promptly notify the health department, even if the diagnosis of Hib disease is only suspected, so it can track the situation and make appropriate decisions about prophylaxis.
- Household members and children who are under-immunized or unimmunized and attending a group care setting where a case of Hib infection has been reported may need to take an antibiotic to prevent the spread of this disease.
- Ensure that exposed children who develop a fever are seen by a health professional as soon as possible.
- Practice careful and frequent hand washing.
- Clean and sanitize surface areas and items that are mouthed by children.
- Avoid sharing food and drinks.

Exclude from group setting?

Yes.
- Exclude all children with proven Hib infection until treatment is completed.
- Note: Do not exclude exposed children and staff as long as they have no other reasons for exclusion.

Readmit to group setting?

- The child is cleared to return by a health professional or the local health department.
- When the child is able to participate and staff determine that they can care for the child without compromising their ability to care for the health and safety of the other children in the group.

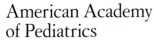

American Academy of Pediatrics

DEDICATED TO THE HEALTH OF ALL CHILDREN™

The American Academy of Pediatrics is an organization of 60,000 primary care pediatricians, pediatric medical subspecialists, and pediatric surgical specialists dedicated to the health, safety, and well-being of infants, children, adolescents, and young adults.

American Academy of Pediatrics
PO Box 747
Elk Grove Village, IL 60009-0747
Web site—http://www.aap.org

Hand-Foot-and-Mouth Disease (Most Commonly Enterovirus)

What is hand-foot-and-mouth disease?

A common viral infection that causes outbreaks of the disease in the summer and fall. Despite its scary name, this illness generally is mild.

What are the signs or symptoms?

- Tiny blisters in the mouth and on the fingers, palms of hands, buttocks, and soles of feet that last a little longer than a week (one, few, or all of these may be present).
- May see common cold signs or symptoms with fever, sore throat, runny nose, and cough. The most troublesome finding often are the blisters in the mouth, which make it difficult for the child to eat or drink. Other signs or symptoms such as vomiting and diarrhea can occur, but are less frequently troublesome.

What are the incubation and contagious periods?

- Incubation period: 3 to 6 days.
- Contagious period: Virus may be shed for several weeks after the infection starts; respiratory shedding of the virus is usually limited to a week or less.

How is it spread?

- Respiratory route (ie, coughing, sneezing)
- Direct contact
- Fecal-oral route

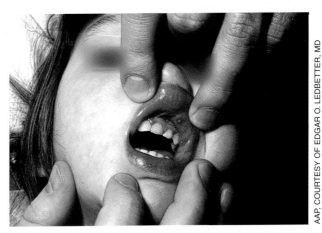

AAP, COURTESY OF EDGAR O. LEDBETTER, MD

Child with blisters inside lips

How do you control it?

- Teach children and caregivers/teachers to cover their mouths and noses when sneezing or coughing with a disposable facial tissue if possible, or with a shoulder if no facial tissue is available in time ("give your cough or sneeze a cold shoulder"). Teach everyone to wash hands right after using facial tissues or having contact with mucus and to change or cover contaminated clothing to prevent the spread of disease by contaminated hands.
- Dispose of facial tissues that contain nasal secretions after each use.
- Practice good hand washing, especially after diaper changing.

What are the roles of the caregiver/teacher and the family?

- Report the infection to staff designated by the child care program or school for decision making and action related to care of ill children. That person, in turn, alerts possibly exposed family members and staff to watch for symptoms.
- Encourage the family to seek medical advice if the child is very uncomfortable with signs of illness from the infection, such as an inability to drink or eat, or if the child seems very ill.

➤ *continued*

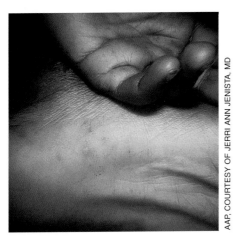

AAP, COURTESY OF JERRI ANN JENISTA, MD

Child with blisters on hands and feet

Hand-Foot-and-Mouth Disease (Most Commonly Enterovirus), continued

Exclude from group setting?

No, unless

- The child is unable to participate and staff determine that they cannot care for the child without compromising their ability to care for the health and safety of the other children in the group.
- The child meets other exclusion criteria, such as fever with behavior change (see "Conditions Requiring Temporary Exclusion" on page 28).
- Note: Exclusion will not reduce disease transmission because some children may shed the virus without becoming recognizably ill, and the virus may be shed for weeks in the stool after the child seems well.

Readmit to group setting?

When exclusion criteria are resolved, the child is able to participate, and staff determine that they can care for the child without compromising their ability to care for the health and safety of the other children in the group

American Academy of Pediatrics

DEDICATED TO THE HEALTH OF ALL CHILDREN™

The American Academy of Pediatrics is an organization of 60,000 primary care pediatricians, pediatric medical subspecialists, and pediatric surgical specialists dedicated to the health, safety, and well-being of infants, children, adolescents, and young adults.

American Academy of Pediatrics
PO Box 747
Elk Grove Village, IL 60009-0747
Web site—http://www.aap.org

Head Lice (Pediculosis Capitis)

What are head lice?

- Small, tan-colored insects (less than $\frac{1}{8}$" long) that
  - ~ Live on blood they draw from the scalp.
  - ~ Crawl (they do not hop or fly).
  - ~ Deposit tiny, gray/white eggs known as *nits* on a hair shaft 3 to 4 mm from the scalp because the eggs need the warmth from the scalp for hatching.
  - ~ Can live only 1 to 2 days away from the scalp.
- Having an infestation with lice may cause irritation and scratching with secondary skin infection.
- Families and caregivers/teachers often get very upset about lice; however, lice do not cause disease. Head lice infestations occur in all socioeconomic groups and do not represent poor hygiene.
- Often, normal activities are disrupted because of excessive reaction to these insect pests.

What are the signs or symptoms?

- Itching of skin where lice feed on the scalp or neck.
- Nits may be glued to hair, commonly behind ears and at or near the nape of the neck.
- Scratching, especially behind and around ears and at the nape of the neck.
- Open sores and crusting from secondary bacterial infection that may be associated with swollen lymph nodes (commonly called *swollen glands*).

What are the incubation and contagious periods?

- Incubation period: 6 to 10 days from laying to hatching of eggs.
  - ~ Lice can reproduce 2 to 3 weeks after hatching.
- Contagious period: Until treated with a chemical that kills lice and viable eggs have been killed or removed.

How are they spread?

- Direct contact with hair or head gear of infected people
- Storing or sharing combs, brushes, hats, blankets, or sheets
- Can spread only by crawling lice (not nits)

How do you control them?

- Pesticides that kill lice and most viable eggs are available. Resistance of lice and nits to these chemicals has been reported, but the extent of resistance to the chemicals is not known. Repeated use of the recommended treatment chemicals to get rid of lice may be more of a safety risk

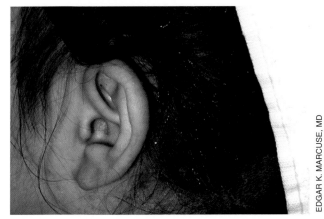

EDGAR K. MARCUSE, MD

Child with nits on hair behind ears and at nape of neck

than lice themselves. Most of these chemicals are potentially toxic with repeated use or misuse.
- None of the suggested remedies using common household products (eg, salad oils, mayonnaise, petroleum jelly) or chemicals intended for other purposes have been shown to be effective. Some that have been tried (eg, kerosene) are very dangerous.
- Mechanical removal of the lice and nits by combing them out with a special fine-tooth comb is tedious and very time consuming. Although such combing is not necessary after using a recommended pediculicide chemical, it helps find lice in the hair and removes the dead nits so that reinfestation of a treated child is easier to detect.
- Examine the heads of household and close contacts using special lice combs, available from drug stores and on the Internet, or use small flat wooden sticks to separate the hair (eg, Popsicle sticks or tongue depressors).
- Articles that may have been contaminated should be laundered so that the fabric is exposed to a temperature of 130°F. Using hot water in a washer and drying on the hot setting kills lice in bedding and clothing. Dry-cleaning clothing and bedding also is effective.
- Toys, personal articles, bedding, other fabrics, and upholstered furniture that cannot be laundered with hot water and a dryer or dry-cleaned can be kept in a plastic bag for 10 days if there is concern about lice having crawled from an infested child onto these articles.
- Because head lice can only live for 1 to 2 days away from the scalp, chemical treatment of the environment is not necessary. Vacuum floors, carpets, mattresses, and furniture (a safe alternative to spraying).

➤ *continued*

Head Lice (Pediculosis Capitis), continued

- Prevent lice infestation.
  - ~ Encourage children not to share headgear, towels, and bedding.
  - ~ Soak combs and brushes in disinfectant solution (¼-cup bleach to 1 gallon of water) for at least 10 minutes. Soaking in pediculicide shampoo or hot water (130°F) for 5 minutes also works.
  - ~ Provide separate storage areas for each child's clothing so that the personal articles of one child do not touch the personal articles of another child (eg, widely placed hooks, non-touching laundry or plastic bags for personal items).

What are the roles of the caregiver/teacher and the family?

- Report the infection to staff designated by the child care program or school for decision making and action related to care of ill children. That person, in turn, alerts possibly exposed family members and staff to watch for symptoms.
- Have parents/guardians consult with a health professional for a treatment plan.
- Check children observed scratching their heads for lice; check all contacts.
- Educate caregivers/teachers and families how to recognize lice and nits.
- Implement other control measures listed here.

Exclude from group setting?

Yes, at the end of the program or school day.

- Children with lice should be referred for treatment at the end of the day.
- Until the end of the program or school day, avoid any activity that involves the child in head-to-head contact with other children or sharing of any headgear.

Readmit to group setting?

After the child has received the treatment recommended by the child's health professional

Comments

- No-nit policies requiring children to be nit-free are not recommended because they may keep the child out of the program needlessly and unduly burden the child's parents/guardians who must implement this measure. Differences of opinion about no-nit policies are common.
- Education of families and caregivers/teachers about the relatively benign consequences of head lice infestations should be attempted to reduce the level of disruption for the infested child and all the others involved in the program. It may be necessary to arrange for a health professional to provide this education to overcome the widespread beliefs about this problem.

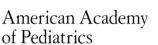

American Academy of Pediatrics

DEDICATED TO THE HEALTH OF ALL CHILDREN™

The American Academy of Pediatrics is an organization of 60,000 primary care pediatricians, pediatric medical subspecialists, and pediatric surgical specialists dedicated to the health, safety, and well-being of infants, children, adolescents, and young adults.

American Academy of Pediatrics
PO Box 747
Elk Grove Village, IL 60009-0747
Web site—http://www.aap.org

Hepatitis A

What is hepatitis A?

- A viral infection causing liver inflammation
- An acute, usually self-limited illness

What are the signs or symptoms?

- Fever.
- Jaundice (ie, yellowing of skin or whites of eyes).
- Abdominal discomfort.
- Tiredness.
- Dark-brown urine.
- Loss of appetite, nausea.
- Children younger than 6 years usually have few or no signs or symptoms.

What are the incubation and contagious periods?

- Incubation period: 15 to 50 days with an average of 25 to 30 days.
- Contagious period: Most infectious in the 2 weeks before onset of signs or symptoms; the risk for transmission is minimal 1 week after onset of jaundice.

How is it spread?

Fecal-oral route

How do you control it?

- Hepatitis A vaccine (for children 2 years and older) in situations and areas of the country where benefits justify cost of the vaccine (ie, communities where hepatitis A disease is widespread).
- In an outbreak situation, immune globulin shots may be recommended by a health department for contacts.
- Good hand washing techniques, especially after diaper changing.
- Child care and school settings have been found to play a significant role in the community-wide spread of hepatitis A. Because young children usually have few or no signs or symptoms, dissemination to adults occurs via contact with children either directly in the group care setting or who are enrolled in a group care setting and then expose adults at home.

What are the roles of the caregiver/teacher and the family?

- Report the infection to staff designated by the child care program or school for decision making and action related to care of ill children. That person, in turn, alerts possibly exposed family members and staff to watch for symptoms.
- Practice good hand washing and hygiene, with special attention to good technique after helping child with toileting or changing diapers.
- Teach children to wash their hands after using the toilet and before any activity potentially involving food or the mouth.
- Clean and sanitize surfaces in all areas. Hepatitis A virus can survive on surfaces for weeks.
- Contact a health professional promptly to review the need for using immune globulin.
- When hepatitis A virus infection is identified in a staff member, child, or the household contacts of 2 or more enrolled children in the group care setting in which children are not toilet trained, immune globulin is recommended for all previously unimmunized staff and children in the facility.
- Depending on when a hepatitis A outbreak is recognized in the group setting and the number of children involved, immune globulin may be indicated not only for children and staff but household members of all attendees, as well.

Exclude from group setting?

Yes.

- Children with the disease should be excluded for 1 week after onset of illness.
- Adults with the illness, especially those who work as food handlers, should be excluded for 1 week after onset of illness.
- Refer to health professional.

Readmit to group setting?

- 1 week after onset of illness and after immune globulin has been given to all contacts
- When the child is able to participate and staff determine that they can care for the child without compromising their ability to care for the health and safety of the other children in the group

➤ *continued*

Hepatitis A, continued

Comments

- Once signs or symptoms of hepatitis A occur, the only treatment is supportive care.
- In the United States, hepatitis A is one of the most commonly reported vaccine-preventable diseases. In some communities where hepatitis A is known to be occurring at a high level, universal use of hepatitis A vaccine is recommended. Because hepatitis A is very common in developing countries, hepatitis A vaccine is recommended for travelers to these countries. Families who do such traveling should be expected to get the vaccine to prevent their children from infecting others on their return to the group care setting.

American Academy
of Pediatrics

DEDICATED TO THE HEALTH OF ALL CHILDREN™

The American Academy of Pediatrics is an organization of 60,000 primary care pediatricians, pediatric medical subspecialists, and pediatric surgical specialists dedicated to the health, safety, and well-being of infants, children, adolescents, and young adults.

American Academy of Pediatrics
PO Box 747
Elk Grove Village, IL 60009-0747
Web site—http://www.aap.org

Hepatitis B

What is hepatitis B?

- A viral infection causing liver inflammation.
- Hepatitis B can lead to serious illness, lifelong infection, liver failure, and liver cancer.

What are the signs or symptoms?

- Flu-like (eg, muscle aches, nausea, vomiting).
- Jaundice (ie, yellowing of skin or whites of eyes, dark urine).
- Loss of appetite.
- Joint pains.
- Tiredness.
- Young children may show few or no signs or symptoms.
- Some people recover fully, but some carry the virus in their blood for a lifetime. Age at the time of infection is a major factor in progression to chronic infection.

What are the incubation and contagious periods?

- Incubation period: 45 to 160 days, with an average of 90 days
- Contagious period: As long as the virus is present in the blood of the infected person (can be for the lifetime of the infected individual)

How is it spread?

- Most commonly through
  ~ Blood or blood products.
  ~ Sexual contact.
- Less commonly through
  ~ Saliva.
  ~ Contact with open sores or the fluid that comes from open sores (wound exudate).
  ~ Direct exposure to blood after injury, bites, or scratches that caused a skin break introducing blood or body fluids from a carrier to another person.
- Hepatitis B virus can remain contagious on surfaces for 7 days.

How do you control it?

- Hepatitis B is a vaccine-preventable disease. Infants should receive vaccine at or soon after birth, with additional doses of the vaccine according to the routine immunization schedule.
- Cover open wounds or sores.
- Follow standard precautions and sanitize surfaces that may have been contaminated with blood, bloody fluids, or other body fluids using a freshly made spray solution of household bleach of 1:64 (1 tablespoon of household bleach in 1 quart of water, sprayed to wet the surface to glistening, and then left in contact with the surface for at least 2 minutes, or a 1:10 dilution applied with a cloth). Note that standard precautions include universal precautions. Universal precautions is a term used most commonly by the Occupational Safety and Health Administration (OSHA) to cover situations involving blood-borne pathogens in body fluids that contain blood-borne germs. Standard precautions cover situations that involve any type of body fluid, except tears.

What are the roles of the caregiver/teacher and the family?

- Report the infection to the health department, as the health professional who makes the diagnosis may not report that the child who has the infection is a participant in a child care program or school, and this could lead to precious time for controlling the spread of the disease being lost.
- Routinely check that children complete hepatitis B vaccine series according to the most recent recommendations.
- Practice standard precautions (and OSHA universal precautions) for handling blood and other body fluids at all times, as carriers of this infection may not be identified to staff.
- Contact the infected child's health professional for a treatment plan.

Exclude from group setting?

Yes, if

A child with known hepatitis B exhibits any of the following:
- Weeping sores that cannot be covered.
- Biting or scratching behavior.
- A bleeding problem.
- Generalized dermatitis that may produce wounds or weepy tissue fluids.
- The child meets other exclusion criteria, such as fever with behavior change (see "Conditions Requiring Temporary Exclusion" on page 28).

➤ *continued*

Hepatitis B, continued

Readmit to group setting?

- When skin lesions are dry or covered
- When the child is cleared to return by a health professional
- When the child is able to participate and staff determine that they can care for the child without compromising their ability to care for the health and safety of the other children in the group

Comments

- Risk of hepatitis B transmission in child care and schools is very small.
- A health professional and staff who the program has designated for decision making and action related to care of ill children need to assess admission of a hepatitis B carrier on an individual basis. Some children who are hepatitis B positive may be in child care or schools, unknown to the health professional, caregivers/teachers, and families. If a child is known to be a hepatitis B carrier, the major issues that determine admission are
  - ~ Dermatitis or bleeding problem
  - ~ Aggressive behavior, including biting

- Hepatitis C also is transmitted through blood and causes a disease similar to hepatitis B. It should be managed the same as hepatitis B.
- Hepatitis D also is transmitted through the blood, but only occurs in those previously infected with hepatitis B. Hepatitis D can be a more severe disease. It is also managed just like hepatitis B.
- Currently, there is no hepatitis C or hepatitis D vaccine available.

American Academy of Pediatrics

DEDICATED TO THE HEALTH OF ALL CHILDREN™

The American Academy of Pediatrics is an organization of 60,000 primary care pediatricians, pediatric medical subspecialists, and pediatric surgical specialists dedicated to the health, safety, and well-being of infants, children, adolescents, and young adults.

American Academy of Pediatrics
PO Box 747
Elk Grove Village, IL 60009-0747
Web site—http://www.aap.org

Herpes Simplex

What is herpes simplex?

- A virus that can cause a variety of infections in different age groups.
- In early childhood, most commonly causes blister-like sores in the mouth and around the lips and on tissues that are in contact with the mouth, such as a sucked thumb or finger.
- Virus may be shed by people with no signs or symptoms (often by adults).

What are the signs or symptoms?

- Fever.
- Irritability.
- Tender, swollen lymph nodes.
- Painful, small, fluid-filled blisters in the mouth, on the gums, and lips.
- Blisters weep clear fluid and are slow to crust over.

What are the incubation and contagious periods?

- Incubation period: 2 days to 2 weeks.
- Contagious period: During the first infection, people shed the virus for at least a week and occasionally for several weeks after signs or symptoms appear. After the first infection, the virus may be reactivated from time to time, producing cold sores in a small number of people. People with recurrent infections shed the largest amount of virus for 3 to 4 days after signs or symptoms appear. Virus shedding may occur at lower levels when infected individuals have no signs or symptoms.

How is it spread?

- Direct contact through kissing and contact with open sores
- Contact with saliva (eg, from mouthed toys)

How do you control it?

- Exercise careful and frequent hand washing.
- Avoid kissing or nuzzling children when a cold sore is present.
- Do not share food or drinks with children or staff.
- Do not touch sores.
- Avoid the sharing of respiratory secretions through contact with objects.

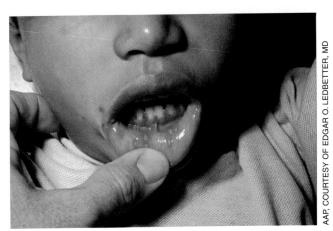

Child with blister-like sores of the mouth and skin around the lips

AAP, COURTESY OF EDGAR O. LEDBETTER, MD

What are the roles of the caregiver/teacher and the family?

- Report the infection to staff designated by the child care program or school for decision making and action related to care of ill children. That person, in turn, alerts possibly exposed family members and staff to watch for symptoms.
- Stress the importance of good hand washing and other measures aimed at controlling the transmission of infected secretions (eg, saliva, tissue fluid, fluid from a skin sore).
- Wash and sanitize mouthed toys, bottle nipples, and utensils that have come into contact with saliva or have been touched by children who are drooling and put fingers in their mouths.
- Avoiding any touching of cold sores with hands is difficult, but should be attempted. When sores have been touched, careful hand washing should follow immediately.

Exclude from group setting?

No, unless

- The child has mouth ulcers and blisters and does not have control of drooling.
- The child is unable to participate and staff determine that they cannot care for the child without compromising their ability to care for the health and safety of the other children in the group.
- The child meets other exclusion criteria, such as fever with behavior change (see "Conditions Requiring Temporary Exclusion" on page 28).

➤ *continued*

Herpes Simplex, continued

- Note: Children and caregivers/teachers with recurrent infection (ie, cold sores) do not need to be excluded but should have sores covered by clothing, adhesive bandages, or dressing if possible.

Readmit to group setting?

- When no drooling or exposed open sores
- When the child is able to participate and staff determine that they can care for the child without compromising their ability to care for the health and safety of the other children in the group

**American Academy
of Pediatrics**

DEDICATED TO THE HEALTH OF ALL CHILDREN™

The American Academy of Pediatrics is an organization of 60,000 primary care pediatricians, pediatric medical subspecialists, and pediatric surgical specialists dedicated to the health, safety, and well-being of infants, children, adolescents, and young adults.

American Academy of Pediatrics
PO Box 747
Elk Grove Village, IL 60009-0747
Web site—http://www.aap.org

Human Immunodeficiency Virus/Acquired Immunodeficiency Syndrome (HIV/AIDS)

What is human immunodeficiency virus/ acquired immunodeficiency syndrome?

An infectious disease caused by a virus that progressively destroys the body's immune system

What are the signs or symptoms?

Children with HIV infection may show few signs or symptoms. Some may have
- Failure to grow and develop well
- Enlarged lymph nodes
- Swelling of salivary glands
- Enlargement of the liver
- Frequent infections, including pneumonia, diarrhea, and thrush (ie, a yeast infection on the surfaces of the mouth)

What are the incubation and contagious periods?

- Incubation period: If the infection is acquired before or during birth from infected mothers, infants typically develop signs or symptoms between 12 and 18 months of age, although some remain symptom-free for more than 5 years.
- Contagious period: Infected individuals can transmit the virus throughout their lifetime.

How is it spread?

- Contact of mucous membranes or openings in the skin with infected blood and body fluids that contain blood, semen, and cervical secretions; also can be spread from mother to infant through breastfeeding.
- Contaminated needles or sharp instruments.
- Mother-infant transmission before or during birth.
- Sexual contact.
- HIV is not spread by the type of contact that occurs in child care and school settings, such as typical classroom activities, or with surfaces touched by infected people. It is not spread through saliva, tears, stool, or urine.

How do you control it?

- Standard precautions should be followed when blood or blood-containing body fluids are handled. For blood and blood-containing substances, these are the same precautions described by the Occupational Safety and Health Administration (OSHA) as universal precautions.
  - ~ Wear disposable or utility gloves that can be sanitized after use.

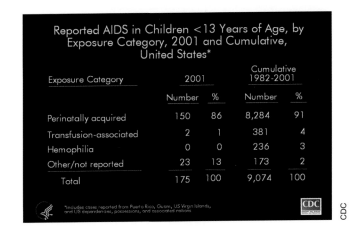

Reported AIDS in Children <13 Years of Age, by Exposure Category, 2001 and Cumulative, United States*

Exposure Category	2001		Cumulative 1982-2001	
	Number	%	Number	%
Perinatally acquired	150	86	8,284	91
Transfusion-associated	2	1	381	4
Hemophilia	0	0	236	3
Other/not reported	23	13	173	2
Total	175	100	9,074	100

*Includes cases reported from Puerto Rico, Guam, US Virgin Islands, and US dependencies, possessions, and associated nations

CDC

- ~ Absorb as much of the spill as possible with disposable materials; put the contaminated materials in a plastic bag with a secure tie.
- ~ Clean contaminated surfaces with detergent, soap, and water.
- ~ Rinse with water.
- ~ Sanitize the clean surface by wetting the entire surface with a spray application of freshly diluted domestic bleach (¼-cup bleach in 1 gallon of water equals 1 tablespoon to a quart) and leaving this solution in contact with the surface for at least 2 minutes.
- ~ Dispose of all soiled items in plastic bags with secure ties.
- Admit children who are known to be infected with HIV whose health status makes their participation acceptable for their health and the health of the others of the group, judged on a case-by-case basis by collaborative decision making involving the program director or school principal and a health professional who is knowledgeable about HIV infection. If the child has one or more potential risk factors for transmission of blood-borne pathogens, such as generalized skin rash or bleeding problems, the child should be assessed by the child's health professional and the child care program director or school principal to see whether the child's risk factors can be managed to allow the child to participate in the program or preclude contact with other children.

What are the roles of the caregiver/teacher and the family?

- Parents/guardians of all children, including children with HIV, should be notified immediately if a case of a highly contagious disease, such as measles or chickenpox, occurs in group care settings.

➤ continued

Human Immunodeficiency Virus/Acquired Immunodeficiency Syndrome (HIV/AIDS), continued

- Parents of children with HIV should consult with their children's health professional when their children have been exposed to a potentially harmful infectious disease.
- All staff in child care and school settings should receive annual education about standard precautions, which include OSHA requirements for universal precautions.
- Parents/guardians do not have to share information about the HIV status of their children. If parents/guardians share HIV status of their children, this information is not to be disclosed to staff without written permission of the parents/guardians.

Exclude from group setting?

No, unless

- The child has fever or behavior change.
- The child has weeping skin lesions that cannot be covered.
- The child has bleeding problems.
- The child meets other exclusion criteria (see "Conditions Requiring Temporary Exclusion" on page 28).

Readmit to group setting?

- A child who is known to have HIV and has been excluded because of risk of exposure to infections in the group care setting can return when the child's health professional determines it is safe for the child to return.
- When skin lesions are dry or covered.
- When the child is able to participate and staff determine that they can care for the child without compromising their ability to care for the health and safety of the other children in the group.

Comment

See *Caring for Our Children,* standards 3.026, 3.027, 6.033, 6.034, 8.053, and 8.057, for more details on HIV/AIDS policies.

American Academy
of Pediatrics

DEDICATED TO THE HEALTH OF ALL CHILDREN™

The American Academy of Pediatrics is an organization of 60,000 primary care pediatricians, pediatric medical subspecialists, and pediatric surgical specialists dedicated to the health, safety, and well-being of infants, children, adolescents, and young adults.

American Academy of Pediatrics
PO Box 747
Elk Grove Village, IL 60009-0747
Web site—http://www.aap.org

Impetigo

What is impetigo?

A common skin infection caused by streptococcal or staphylococcal bacteria

What are the signs or symptoms?

Small, red pimples or fluid-filled blisters with crusted yellow scabs found most often on the face, but may be anywhere on body

What are the incubation and contagious periods?

- Incubation period: Skin sores develop in 7 to 10 days after bacteria attach to the skin.
- Contagious period: Until the skin sores are treated with antibiotics for at least 24 hours or the crusting lesions are no longer present.

How is it spread?

- Direct contact with an infected person or from contaminated surfaces.
- Germ enters an opening on skin (eg, cut, insect bite, burn) and causes oozing, leading to honey-colored crusted sores.
- Occurs year-round, but most common in warm weather in cut and scraped skin. Also occurs in cold weather when the skin around the nose and face is damaged by runny nasal secretions and nose wiping that irritates the skin.

How do you control it?

- Exclusion of infected individuals until antibiotics started for 24 hours.
- Hand washing.
- Clip fingernails to reduce further injury of tissues by scratching and subsequent spread through contaminated fingernails.
- In the event of an outbreak (more than one infected child in a group), consult with the local health department. The problem could involve antibiotic-resistant staphylococcal bacteria.

What are the roles of the caregiver/teacher and the family?

- Consult health professional for a treatment plan.
- Exercise good hand hygiene.
- Clean infected area with soap and water.
- Loosely cover infected area to allow airflow for healing and avoid contact with others in group care settings.
- Wash hands after coming into contact with sores or when changing bandages at the group setting and home.
- Launder contaminated clothing articles daily.
- Notify the local health department if an outbreak occurs.

Exclude from group setting?

Yes.
- As soon as suspected.
- If family is unable to pick up the child promptly, wash affected area with soap and water and cover it.

Readmit to group setting?

- Twenty-four hours after beginning medication
- When the child is able to participate and staff determine that they can care for the child without compromising their ability to care for the health and safety of the other children in the group

Comment

When impetigo is caused by group A streptococcus, treatment and complication issues are similar to when this bacterium causes strep throat (see "Strep Throat (Streptococcal Pharyngitis) and Scarlet Fever").

American Academy of Pediatrics

DEDICATED TO THE HEALTH OF ALL CHILDREN™

The American Academy of Pediatrics is an organization of 60,000 primary care pediatricians, pediatric medical subspecialists, and pediatric surgical specialists dedicated to the health, safety, and well-being of infants, children, adolescents, and young adults.

American Academy of Pediatrics
PO Box 747
Elk Grove Village, IL 60009-0747
Web site—http://www.aap.org

Influenza

What is influenza?

A contagious disease caused by a group of respiratory viruses called the influenza viruses.

What are the signs or symptoms?

- Sudden onset of fever
- Headache
- Chills
- Muscle aches and pains
- Sore throat
- Cough
- Mild pinkeye
- Decreased energy
- Abdominal pain
- Nausea and vomiting (These symptoms alone or with fever often are caused by other factors, not influenza virus.)
- In young infants, croup, bronchiolitis, or pneumonia

What are the incubation and contagious periods?

- Incubation period: 1 to 3 days
- Contagious period: From the day before signs or symptoms appear until 7 days after the onset of flu

How is it spread?

- Direct contact from sneezing and coughing
- Indirect contact from contaminated hands and articles soiled with nose and throat secretions

How do you control it?

- Annual immunization guided by the most recent immunization recommendations.
  - ~ Beginning in 2004, the influenza vaccine is recommended for all children with a high risk of severe illness from influenza disease as well as healthy children 6 to 23 months of age. Children who are 6 to 23 months of age have the highest hospitalization rate of all age groups. Also note that children in group care settings have an increased risk of acquiring influenza compared with children who are not in any type of group care.

The American Academy of Pediatrics (AAP) recommends consideration of influenza immunization for groups of people whose close contact facilitates rapid transmission and spread of infection that may result in disruption of routine activities. These groups include children in child care and school settings.

- Careful and frequent hand washing.
- Teach children and caregivers/teachers to cover their noses and mouths when sneezing or coughing with a disposable facial tissue, if possible, or with a shoulder if no facial tissue is available in time ("give your cough or sneeze a cold shoulder"). Teach everyone to wash their hands right after using facial tissues or having contact with mucus to prevent the spread of disease by contaminated hands and to remove, change, or cover contaminated clothing. Dispose of facial tissues that contain nasal secretions after each use.
- Wash hands after contact with any soiled items.
- Medications that help control viral infections may be helpful if given early in the course of illness.

What are the roles of the caregiver/teacher and the family?

- Follow the AAP recommendation to immunize children at high risk of severe illness from influenza infection, healthy children between 6 and 23 months of age, as well as household contacts and out-of-home caregivers of all children younger than 24 months annually. Also consider annual influenza immunization of all staff and children in group care settings.
- Avoid aspirin use for anyone with influenza; there is an increased risk of Reye syndrome when aspirin is used in this situation.

Exclude from group setting?

No, unless

- The child is unable to participate and staff determine that they cannot care for the child without compromising their ability to care for the health and safety of the other children in the group.
- The child meets other exclusion criteria, such as fever with behavior change (see "Conditions Requiring Temporary Exclusion" on page 28).

➤ *continued*

Influenza, continued

Readmit to group setting?

When exclusion criteria are resolved, the child is able to participate, and staff determine that they can care for the child without compromising their ability to care for the health and safety of the other children in the group

American Academy
of Pediatrics

DEDICATED TO THE HEALTH OF ALL CHILDREN™

The American Academy of Pediatrics is an organization of 60,000 primary care pediatricians, pediatric medical subspecialists, and pediatric surgical specialists dedicated to the health, safety, and well-being of infants, children, adolescents, and young adults.

American Academy of Pediatrics
PO Box 747
Elk Grove Village, IL 60009-0747
Web site—http://www.aap.org

Lyme Disease (and Other Tick-borne Diseases)

What is Lyme disease?

An infection caused by a type of bacteria known as spirochetes that are transmitted when particular types of ticks attach to a person's skin and feed on that person's blood. The common name for this type of tick is the deer tick.

What are the signs or symptoms?

- Gradually expanding, large, circular or oval-shaped rash with a partial central clear area that appears after a tick bite.
- Fever.
- Headache.
- Mild neck stiffness.
- Flu-like signs or symptoms.
- Untreated Lyme disease may lead to arthritis, neurologic problems, or meningitis.

What are the incubation and contagious periods?

- Incubation period: 3 to 31 days from tick bite to appearance of rash.
- Contagious period: Lyme disease is not contagious, except through blood transfusions.

How is it spread?

When infected ticks attach and feed on humans long enough (greater than 36 hours)

How do you control it?

- Avoid tick habitats (eg, tall grassy areas, bushes, wooded areas) if possible. Walk in the center of trails to limit brushing against trees, bushes, and high grasses.
- If children will be in tick-infested areas, dress them with hats, light-colored clothing, long sleeves, long pants tucked into socks, and closed shoes.
- Spray permethrin on clothing to prevent tick attachment. Apply the spray to the clothing when it is off the child in a well-ventilated area outdoors.
- DEET also may be applied to exposed skin according to Centers for Disease Control and Prevention instructions (www.cdc.gov/ncidod/dvbid/westnile/qa/insect_repellent.htm).
  - ~ DEET should not be used in a product that combines the repellent with a sunscreen. Sunscreens often are applied repeatedly because they can be washed off. DEET is not water-soluble and will last up to 8 hours. Repeated application may increase the potential toxic effects of DEET.

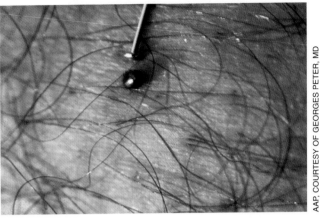

Child with a deer tick attached to skin (compared with the head of a sewing pin)

AAP, COURTESY OF GEORGES PETER, MD

  - ~ When using repellent on a child, adults should apply it to their own hands and then rub them on the child.
  - ~ Apply DEET sparingly on exposed skin; do not use under clothing. If repellent is applied to clothing, wash or dry-clean treated clothing before wearing again.
  - ~ Do not use DEET on the hands of young children; avoid applying to areas around the eyes and mouth.
  - ~ Do not use DEET over cuts, wounds, or irritated skin. Wash treated skin with soap and water after returning indoors; wash treated clothing.
  - ~ Avoid spraying in enclosed areas; do not use DEET near food.
  - ~ Concentrations of 10% to 30% DEET are safe and effective. Ten-percent DEET offers approximately 2 hours of protection, whereas 30% offers at least 5 hours of protection. The concentration of DEET should be tailored to the amount of time the child will be outdoors.
  - ~ Do not use DEET in children younger than 2 months.
  - ~ Treat tick repellent as an over-the-counter medication, obtaining the parent/guardian's written consent and the health professional's written or telephone instructions for use.
- Lyme disease is treatable with antibiotics.

What are the roles of the caregiver/teacher and the family?

- Inspect children's skin and scalps after possible tick exposure.
- For removal, a tick should be grasped with fine tweezers close to the skin and gently pulled straight out without twisting motions. If fingers are used to remove ticks, the skin of the person removing the tick should be protected with facial tissue and washed after tick removal.

➤ *continued*

Lyme Disease (and Other Tick-borne Diseases), continued

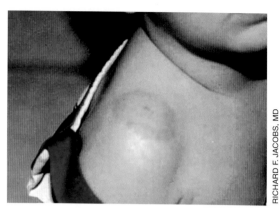

RICHARD F. JACOBS, MD

Child with the rash of Lyme disease at the site of a
tick bite on shoulder

- Be sure to tell parents/guardians that the child has had a
tick bite. The tick usually does not need to be saved for
identification; follow the instructions of public health
officials about the need to save ticks.

Exclude from group setting?

No, unless

- The child is unable to participate and staff determine that
they cannot care for the child without compromising their
ability to care for the health and safety of the other children
in the group.
- The child meets other exclusion criteria, such as fever with
behavior change (see "Conditions Requiring Temporary
Exclusion" on page 28).

Readmit to group setting?

When exclusion criteria are resolved, the child is able to
participate, and staff determine that they can care for the
child without compromising their ability to care for the
health and safety of the other children in the group

Comments

Lyme disease occurs primarily in 3 regions of the
United States.

- Most cases are reported in the Northeast, from southern
Maine to northern Virginia.
- The disease occurs less often in the upper Midwest and
on the West Coast.
- Lyme disease is common (endemic) in at least 10 states.

Other Tick-borne Diseases

Ticks also transmit the following conditions; therefore, control
measures and exclusion and readmission criteria are the same
as for Lyme disease. Note that infected individuals may not be
aware of a recent tick bite. All of these conditions are treatable
with antibiotics.

- Rocky Mountain spotted fever
  - ~ Signs or symptoms: Severe headache, fever, muscle aches,
  nausea, vomiting, and a red, bumpy rash that begins on
  wrists and ankles and proceeds toward the center of the
  body. The illness may be severe or fatal in some cases.
  - ~ Occurs in the south Atlantic, southeastern, and south
  central regions of the United States.
  - ~ Incubation period: 2 to 14 days after dog tick or wood
  tick bite.
- Ehrlichiosis
  - ~ Signs or symptoms: Similar to Rocky Mountain spotted
  fever, except the rash is less common. Less severe than
  Rocky Mountain spotted fever.
  - ~ Occurs primarily in the southeastern and south central
  regions of the United States, but occasionally may occur
  in other regions.
  - ~ Incubation period: 5 to 10 days after deer tick or lone star
  tick bite.
- Tularemia
  - ~ Signs or symptoms: Fever, chills, muscle aches, and
  headache. May involve painful bite site with swollen and
  draining lymph nodes.
  - ~ Occurs from tick or wild animal bites, most commonly
  rabbits.
- Babesiosis
  - ~ Signs or symptoms: Fever, chills or sweats, muscle or
  joint aches, and nausea or vomiting.
  - ~ Transmitted by the same tick that causes Lyme disease.

American Academy
of Pediatrics

DEDICATED TO THE HEALTH OF ALL CHILDREN™

The American Academy of Pediatrics is an organization of 60,000 primary care pediatricians, pediatric medical subspecialists, and pediatric surgical
specialists dedicated to the health, safety, and well-being of infants, children, adolescents, and young adults.

American Academy of Pediatrics
PO Box 747
Elk Grove Village, IL 60009-0747
Web site—http://www.aap.org

Measles

What is measles?

- A highly contagious and acute viral disease caused by the measles virus. Humans are the only natural host for the measles virus.
- Very infrequent in the United States among individuals with adequate immunizations (or those who are old enough to have had the disease before vaccine was available). Outbreaks continue to occur among those who have not been protected by the vaccine.

What are the signs or symptoms?

- Fever, cough, runny nose, and red, watery eyes.
- Small red spots in mouth (called Koplik spots).
- Appearance of rash at hairline spreading downward over body.
- May have diarrhea or ear infection.
- Complications may be serious and result in pneumonia, brain inflammation, convulsions, deafness, or mental retardation.

What are the incubation and contagious periods?

- Incubation period: 8 to 12 days from exposure to onset of signs or symptoms
- Contagious period: From 1 to 2 days before the first signs or symptoms appear (3 to 5 days before the rash) until 4 days after the appearance of the rash

How is it spread?

Direct contact with respiratory droplets

How do you control it?

- Measles, mumps, and rubella (MMR) vaccine, according to the most recent immunization recommendations. Review immunization status of all children and staff.
- For outbreaks, exclude exposed children who have not been immunized until they become immunized or, if they are not immunized because of an accepted exemption from immunization, continue to exclude them until the health department determines it is safe for them to return.
- Hand washing and routine infection control measures.

What are the roles of the caregiver/teacher and the family?

- Report the infection to staff designated by the child care program or school for decision making and action related to care of ill children. That person, in turn, alerts possibly exposed family members and staff to watch for symptoms.
- Report the infection to the health department, as the health professional who makes the diagnosis may not report that the child who has the infection is a participant in a child care program or school, and this could lead to precious time for controlling the spread of the disease being lost.
- Review and ensure that all children have received MMR vaccine according to current immunization recommendations.
- Ensure that staff members who have had less than 2 doses of vaccine are properly immunized, unless documented to have had the disease or were born before 1957 (presumed immune).
- Exclude exposed children with weakened immune systems and who have not received MMR vaccine.

Exclude from group setting?

Yes.

- Measles is a highly communicable illness for which routine exclusion of infected children is warranted.
- Unimmunized people who have been exempted from measles immunization for medical, religious, or other reasons, if not immunized within 72 hours of exposure, should be excluded from the group care setting until at least 2 weeks after the onset of rash in the last case of measles.

Readmit to group setting?

- Four days after beginning of rash
- When the child is able to participate and staff determine that they can care for the child without compromising their ability to care for the health and safety of the other children in the group

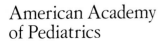

American Academy of Pediatrics

DEDICATED TO THE HEALTH OF ALL CHILDREN™

The American Academy of Pediatrics is an organization of 60,000 primary care pediatricians, pediatric medical subspecialists, and pediatric surgical specialists dedicated to the health, safety, and well-being of infants, children, adolescents, and young adults.

American Academy of Pediatrics
PO Box 747
Elk Grove Village, IL 60009-0747
Web site—http://www.aap.org

Meningitis

What is meningitis?

- An infectious disease causing swelling or inflammation of the tissue covering the spinal cord and brain.
- Three types of bacteria most commonly cause bacterial meningitis in young children.
  - ~ Meningococcus
  - ~ Pneumococcus
  - ~ *Haemophilus influenzae* type b (Hib)
- With current immunization, meningitis from the pneumococcus bacteria is uncommon and from Hib is rare.
- Most commonly caused by viruses. Although most cases of viral meningitis resolve without antimicrobial treatment or complications, it can be confused with bacterial meningitis in early stages.
- Viral meningitis typically occurs during summer and early fall in temperate climates.
- Viral meningitis in young infants can cause neurologic/developmental problems in a small percentage of cases.

What are the signs or symptoms?

- Fever (may be associated with a bloodred rash of meningococcus)
- Headache
- Nausea
- Loss of appetite
- Sometimes a stiff neck (ie, pain or discomfort when trying to touch the chin to the chest; child is unwilling to bend head forward enough to look at her/his "belly button")
- Irritability
- Photophobia (ie, discomfort when looking into bright lights)
- Confusion
- Drowsiness
- Seizures
- Coma

What are the incubation and contagious periods?

- Incubation period
  - ~ For the most common cause of viral meningitis (enterovirus): 3 to 6 days
  - ~ For Hib: Unknown
  - ~ For meningococcus and pneumococcus: Less than 4 days
- Contagious period
  - ~ For enterovirus viral meningitis: Shedding of the virus in feces can continue for several weeks, but shedding from the respiratory tract usually lasts a week or less.
  - ~ For Hib, meningococcus, and pneumococcus: Until after 24 hours of antibiotics.

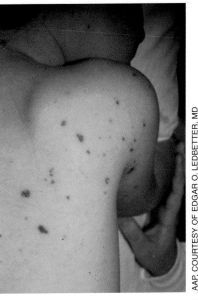

AAP, COURTESY OF EDGAR O. LEDBETTER, MD

Toddler with the rash of meningococcus infection

How is it spread?

- Direct contact with respiratory secretions
- Fecal-oral route (enterovirus)

How do you control it?

- Bacterial meningitis
  - ~ Immunizations according to the latest recommendations.
  - ~ Antibiotic prophylaxis may be indicated for close contacts.
  - ~ Vaccinate unimmunized or under-immunized children as indicated by local health department.
- Viral meningitis
  - ~ Hand washing
  - ~ Routine infection control measures
  - ~ Immunization according to the current universal schedule recommended by the American Academy of Pediatrics, Advisory Committee on Immunization Practices, and American Academy of Family Physicians

What are the roles of the caregiver/teacher and the family?

- Report the infection to staff designated by the child care program or school for decision making and action related to care of ill children. That person, in turn, alerts possibly exposed family members and staff to watch for symptoms.

➤ *continued*

Meningitis, continued

- Report the infection to the health department, as the health professional who makes the diagnosis may not report that the child who has the infection is a participant in a child care program or school, and this could lead to loss of precious time for controlling the spread of the disease.
- Distinguish between viral and bacterial meningitis.
- If it is bacterial meningitis, contact the health professional or health department to see if preventive antibiotic treatment is appropriate for children who have been in contact with the ill child.
- Teach children and caregivers/teachers to cover their noses and mouths when sneezing or coughing with a disposable facial tissue if possible, or with a shoulder if no facial tissue is available in time ("give your cough or sneeze a cold shoulder"). Teach everyone to remove any soil, change or cover contaminated clothing, and wash their hands right after using facial tissues or having contact with mucus to prevent the spread of disease by contaminated hands.
- Dispose of facial tissues that contain nasal secretions after each use.
- Practice good hand hygiene.

Exclude from group setting?

Yes, as soon as it is suspected.

Readmit to group setting?

- When the child is cleared to return by a health professional
- When the child is able to participate and staff determine that they can care for the child without compromising their ability to care for the health and safety of the other children in the group

Molluscum Contagiosum

What is molluscum contagiosum?

A skin disease caused by a virus, somewhat similar to warts

What are the signs or symptoms?

Small, flesh-colored bumps on the skin, often with a tiny, hard, indented, seed-like center

What are the incubation and contagious periods?

- Incubation period: Usually between 2 and 7 weeks, but may be as long as 6 months
- Contagious period: Unknown

How is it spread?

- Person-to-person through close contact
- Through inanimate objects such as towels

How do you control it?

- Wash hands after touching the bumps.
- Do not share towels used by an infected child or adult.
- Scratching the bumps may cause further spread of the virus to another site.
- Usually goes away on its own in a few months as the person develops antibodies to the virus.
- Alternatively, treatments may be used; however, there is little agreement on effective treatments.
- Although molluscum contagiosum bumps represent a viral infection, they are very mildly contagious and most often are spread to other areas of the affected child's body, rather than to other children. Molluscum contagiosum bumps do not need to be covered like shingles or other oozing sores. Treatment is a personal choice and not an infection control issue for a group care setting.

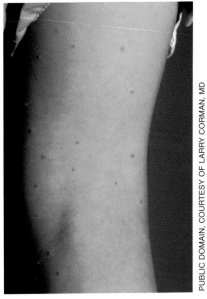

PUBLIC DOMAIN, COURTESY OF LARRY CORMAN, MD

Child with the very small, firm bumps of molluscum contagiosum on back of thigh and knee

What are the roles of the caregiver/teacher and the family?

- Practice careful and frequent hand washing after contact with the bumps.
- Do not let children pick at their bumps because this may cause an opening in the skin, which promotes bacterial infection.

Exclude from group setting?

No.

Comments

This infection can be itchy and spread by children who scratch the bumps and then touch other surfaces and people. This type of itch can be nearly eliminated by applying a cold compress. Instead of telling children not to scratch, keep a small plastic bag of ice in the freezer with a paper towel to wrap around the ice. Give the wrapped ice bag to children to apply to any area that feels itchy.

American Academy of Pediatrics

DEDICATED TO THE HEALTH OF ALL CHILDREN™

The American Academy of Pediatrics is an organization of 60,000 primary care pediatricians, pediatric medical subspecialists, and pediatric surgical specialists dedicated to the health, safety, and well-being of infants, children, adolescents, and young adults.

American Academy of Pediatrics
PO Box 747
Elk Grove Village, IL 60009-0747
Web site—http://www.aap.org

Mononucleosis

What is mononucleosis?

A disease caused by the Epstein-Barr virus, commonly known as "mono"

What are the signs or symptoms?

- Usually mild or no signs or symptoms in young children.
- Fever.
- Sore throat.
- Fatigue.
- Swollen lymph nodes.
- Rash may occur with those treated with ampicillin or other penicillins.

What are the incubation and contagious periods?

- Incubation period: Estimated to be 30 to 50 days.
- Contagious period: Virus is excreted for many months after infection and can occur intermittently throughout life. The period of communicability is unknown.

How is it spread?

Person-to-person contact
- Kissing on the mouth
- Sharing objects contaminated with saliva (eg, toys, tooth-brushes, cups, bottles)
- May be spread by blood transfusion

How do you control it?

- Hand washing.
- Avoiding sharing of respiratory secretions directly or through contact with objects.
- People with signs and symptoms of mononucleosis should not donate blood or prepare food for others.

What are the roles of the caregiver/teacher and the family?

- Use good hand washing technique at all the times listed in "When to Wash Hands" on page 17.
- Clean and sanitize toys and utensils before they are shared (ie, after each child has used them).
- Ensure that all children have their own toothbrushes, cups, and eating utensils.
- Avoid kissing children on the mouth.

Exclude from group setting?

No, unless
- The child is unable to participate and staff determine that they cannot care for the child without compromising their ability to care for the health and safety of the other children in the group.
- The child meets other exclusion criteria, such as fever with behavior change (see "Conditions Requiring Temporary Exclusion" on page 28).

Readmit to group setting?

When exclusion criteria are resolved, the child is able to participate, and staff determine that they can care for the child without compromising their ability to care for the health and safety of the other children in the group

Comments

- Most people get the infection in early childhood when signs or symptoms are mild and disease goes undiagnosed. However, rarely, the disease can be severe.
- General exclusion of those with mononucleosis is not practical.

American Academy of Pediatrics

DEDICATED TO THE HEALTH OF ALL CHILDREN™

The American Academy of Pediatrics is an organization of 60,000 primary care pediatricians, pediatric medical subspecialists, and pediatric surgical specialists dedicated to the health, safety, and well-being of infants, children, adolescents, and young adults.

American Academy of Pediatrics
PO Box 747
Elk Grove Village, IL 60009-0747
Web site—http://www.aap.org

Mosquito-borne Diseases

What are mosquito-borne diseases?

- Viral diseases spread by infected mosquitoes.
- Examples of such viruses include West Nile virus, eastern equine encephalomyelitis (EEE), St Louis encephalitis (SLE), La Crosse encephalitis, and western equine encephalomyelitis (WEE).
- West Nile virus and EEE are discussed in greater detail because they get the most media attention; however, in children, most of these infections produce no signs or symptoms or mild headache and fever. While 80% of those infected with West Nile virus show no signs or symptoms, in 2003, nearly three fourths of the more than 4,000 cases of West Nile disease reported in the United States had disease of the nervous system. In outbreaks, more severe illness may occur, especially among adults.

What are the signs or symptoms?

- Fever
- Headache
- Body aches
- Nausea
- Vomiting
- Rash
- Convulsions
- Coma
- Paralysis (In West Nile disease, paralysis of the facial muscles [Bell palsy] has been noted.)

What are the incubation and contagious periods?

- Incubation periods
  - ~ West Nile virus   5 to 15 days
  - ~ EEE   3 to 10 days
  - ~ SLE   4 to 14 days
  - ~ La Crosse encephalitis   5 to 15 days
  - ~ WEE   2 to 10 days
- Contagious period: These infections are not contagious.

How are they spread?

Through the bite of an infected mosquito. West Nile disease may be spread by blood transfusion also.

How do you control them?

By avoiding mosquito bites.

- Use insect repellents containing DEET.
  - ~ DEET should not be used in a product that combines the repellent with a sunscreen. Sunscreens often are applied repeatedly because they can be washed off. DEET is not water-soluble and will last up to 8 hours. Repeated application may increase the potential toxic effects of DEET.
  - ~ When using repellent on a child, adults should apply it to their own hands and then rub them on the child.
  - ~ Apply DEET sparingly on exposed skin; do not use under clothing. If repellent is applied to clothing, wash or dry-clean treated clothing before wearing again.
  - ~ Do not use DEET on the hands of young children; avoid applying to areas around the eyes and mouth.
  - ~ Do not use DEET over cuts, wounds, or irritated skin. Wash treated skin with soap and water after returning indoors; wash treated clothing.
  - ~ Avoid spraying in enclosed areas; do not use DEET near food.
  - ~ Concentrations of 10% to 30% DEET are safe and effective. Ten-percent DEET offers approximately 2 hours of protection, whereas 30% offers at least 5 hours of protection. The concentration of DEET should be tailored to the amount of time the child will be outdoors.
  - ~ Do not use DEET in children younger than 2 months.
- Stay inside during dusk and dawn, when mosquitoes are most active. When outside at these times, wear long sleeves and pants.
- Check windows to make sure there are no holes in the screens to allow mosquitoes to get indoors.
- Empty standing water from wading pools, buckets, pet dishes, flowerpots, and other sources that can attract mosquitoes.

What are the roles of the caregiver/teacher and the family?

- Follow public health recommendations about preventing mosquito bites.
- Share information about the disease.

➤ continued

Mosquito-borne Diseases, continued

Exclude from group setting?

No, unless

- The child is unable to participate and staff determine that they cannot care for the child without compromising their ability to care for the health and safety of the other children in the group.
- The child meets other exclusion criteria, such as fever with behavior change (see "Conditions Requiring Temporary Exclusion" on page 28).

Readmit to group setting?

When exclusion criteria are resolved, the child is able to participate, and staff determine that they can care for the child without compromising their ability to care for the health and safety of the other children in the group

Comments

- Mosquitoes become infected with West Nile virus after biting infected birds. If you find a dead bird, report it to your local health department and ask for instructions on disposing of the body. Do not handle the body with your bare hands.
- Most cases of West Nile virus in children are very mild.
- Since 1964, there have been only 4 confirmed cases of EEE per year on average, with a range from 0 to 14 cases per year. However, EEE is the most severe encephalitis.
- States with the largest number of EEE cases are Florida, Georgia, Massachusetts, and New Jersey.
- More common and widespread cases of encephalitis are La Crosse and SLE.

American Academy
of Pediatrics

DEDICATED TO THE HEALTH OF ALL CHILDREN™

The American Academy of Pediatrics is an organization of 60,000 primary care pediatricians, pediatric medical subspecialists, and pediatric surgical specialists dedicated to the health, safety, and well-being of infants, children, adolescents, and young adults.

American Academy of Pediatrics
PO Box 747
Elk Grove Village, IL 60009-0747
Web site—http://www.aap.org

Mumps

What is mumps?

- A viral illness with swelling of one or more of the salivary glands
- Uncommon in children with up-to-date measles, mumps, and rubella (MMR) immunization

What are the signs or symptoms?

- Swollen glands in front of and below the ear, or under the jaw (no swelling or symptoms in one third of infections).
- Fever.
- Headache.
- Earache.
- In teenage boys, painful swelling of the testicles may occur. Girls may have swelling of the ovaries, which may cause abdominal pain.
- Complications include meningitis, deafness (usually permanent), and inflammation of joints.
- Infection during pregnancy may kill or severely harm the fetus.

What are the incubation and contagious periods?

- Incubation period: 16 to 18 days
- Contagious period: From 1 to 2 days before to 5 days after swelling of glands, although virus can be isolated from saliva from 7 days before to 9 days after swelling of glands

How is it spread?

Direct contact with mouth or nose secretions

How do you control it?

- Measles, mumps, and rubella vaccine according to most recent recommendations.
- Review immunization status of all children.

What are the roles of the caregiver/teacher and the family?

- Report the infection to staff designated by the child care program or school for decision making and action related to care of ill children. That person, in turn, alerts possibly exposed family members and staff to watch for symptoms.

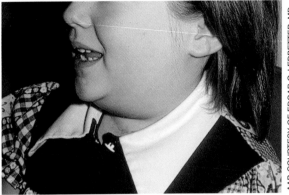

AAP, COURTESY OF EDGAR O. LEDBETTER, MD

Child with swelling around the jaw from mumps

- Report the infection to the health department, as the health professional who makes the diagnosis may not report that the child who has the infection is a participant in a child care program or school, and this could lead to precious time for controlling the spread of the disease being lost.
- Refer to health professional.
- Ensure up-to-date immunization of children, staff, volunteers, and family members with MMR vaccine according to current recommendations.

Exclude from group setting?

Yes.

- Mumps is a highly communicable illness for which routine exclusion of infected children is warranted.
- For outbreaks, exclude exposed children who have not been immunized until they become immunized or, if they are not immunized because of an accepted exemption, continue to exclude them until the health department determines it is safe for them to return.

Readmit to group setting?

- Nine days after onset of swelling
- When the child is able to participate and staff determine that they can care for the child without compromising their ability to care for the health and safety of the other children in the group

Comment

Most cases now occur in young adults.

American Academy
of Pediatrics

DEDICATED TO THE HEALTH OF ALL CHILDREN™

The American Academy of Pediatrics is an organization of 60,000 primary care pediatricians, pediatric medical subspecialists, and pediatric surgical specialists dedicated to the health, safety, and well-being of infants, children, adolescents, and young adults.

American Academy of Pediatrics
PO Box 747
Elk Grove Village, IL 60009-0747
Web site—http://www.aap.org

Pinkeye (Conjunctivitis)

What is conjunctivitis?

Inflammation (ie, redness, swelling) of the thin tissue covering the white part of the eye and the inside of the eyelids

What are the signs or symptoms?

There are several kinds of conjunctivitis, including

- Bacterial
  - ~ Red or pink, itchy, painful.
  - ~ More than a tiny amount of green or yellow discharge.
  - ~ Infected eyes may be crusted shut in the morning.
  - ~ May affect one or both eyes.
- Viral
  - ~ Pink, swollen, watering eye(s) sensitive to light.
  - ~ May affect only one eye.
- Allergic
  - ~ Itching, redness, and excessive tearing, usually of both eyes.
- Chemical
  - ~ Red, watery eyes, especially after swimming in chlorinated water.

What are the incubation and contagious periods?

Depending on the type of conjunctivitis, incubation period varies.

- Bacterial
  - ~ The incubation period is unknown because the bacteria that cause it are commonly present in most individuals and do not usually cause infection.
  - ~ The contagious period ends when the course of medication is started.
- Viral
  - ~ Sometimes occurs early in the course of a viral respiratory disease that has other signs or symptoms.
  - ~ One type of viral conjunctivitis, adenovirus, may be contagious up to 14 days after the appearance of signs or symptoms.
  - ~ The contagious period continues while the signs or symptoms are present.
- Allergic
  - ~ Occurs in response to contact with the agent that causes the allergic reaction. The reaction may be immediate or delayed for many hours or days after the contact.
  - ~ No contagious period.
- Chemical
  - ~ Usually appears shortly after contact with the irritating substance.
  - ~ No contagious period.

How is it spread?

Hands become contaminated by direct contact with discharge from the infected eye, or by touching other surfaces that have been contaminated by the secretions from the child's eyes.

How do you control it?

- Consult health professional for diagnosis and treatment. Antibiotics are needed only for signs of bacterial conjunctivitis (ie, redness *and* green or yellow discharge).
- Careful hand washing before and after touching the eyes, nose, and mouth.
- Careful sanitation of objects that are commonly touched by hands or faces such as tables, doorknobs, telephones, cots, cuddle blankets, and toys.

What are the roles of the caregiver/teacher and the family?

- Report the infection to staff designated by the child care program or school for decision making and action related to care of ill children. That person, in turn, alerts possibly exposed family members and staff to watch for symptoms.
- Notify child's parent/guardian to consult with the child's health professional about diagnosis and treatment (by telephone or office visit).
- Seek advice from the health department or the program's health consultant about how to prevent further spread if more than 2 children have the infection at the same time.
- Review hand washing techniques and sanitation routines.
- Complete course of medication if indicated for bacterial conjunctivitis.

Exclude from group setting?

- **Yes** for bacterial conjunctivitis (ie, red eyes *and* green or yellow discharge).
- **No** for all other forms, except on recommendation of the health department or the child's health professional for epidemic adenoviral conjunctivitis.

➤ *continued*

Pinkeye (Conjunctivitis), continued

Readmit to group setting?

- After exclusion for bacterial conjunctivitis, the child may return after treatment has begun with antibiotic eye drops or ointment.
- When the child is able to participate and staff determine that they can care for the child without compromising their ability to care for the health and safety of the other children in the group.

Comments

- Although many cases of bacterial conjunctivitis can resolve without antibiotic treatment, the course can be shortened and the chance of spread of infection reduced by treatment with antibiotics.
- One form of viral conjunctivitis, caused by adenovirus, can cause epidemics. If more than 2 children in a group care setting develop conjunctivitis in the same time period, seek the advice of the program's health consultant.

American Academy of Pediatrics

DEDICATED TO THE HEALTH OF ALL CHILDREN™

The American Academy of Pediatrics is an organization of 60,000 primary care pediatricians, pediatric medical subspecialists, and pediatric surgical specialists dedicated to the health, safety, and well-being of infants, children, adolescents, and young adults.

American Academy of Pediatrics
PO Box 747
Elk Grove Village, IL 60009-0747
Web site—http://www.aap.org

Pinworms

What are pinworms?

- Small, white, threadlike worms (0.25"–0.5" long) that live in the large intestine

What are the signs or symptoms?

Itching and irritation around the anal or vaginal area

What are the incubation and contagious periods?

- Incubation period: 1 to 2 months or longer from the time of ingesting the pinworm egg until an adult worm migrates to the anal area
- Contagious period: As long as the female worms are discharging eggs to the skin around the anus

How are they spread?

- Fecal-oral route.
- Directly or indirectly by sharing toys, bedding, clothing, toilet seats, or baths.
- Pinworm eggs remain infective for 2 to 3 weeks in indoor environments.
- Infestation with pinworms commonly clusters within families.

How do you control them?

- Good hand hygiene is the most effective method of prevention.
- Treatment with oral medication once or repeated in 2 weeks may be necessary for the whole family and the group of children who share a common environment.

What are the roles of the caregiver/teacher and the family?

- Report the infection to staff designated by the child care program or school for decision making and action related to care of ill children. That person, in turn, alerts possibly exposed family members and staff to watch for symptoms.
- Suspect pinworms if a child has intense itching around the anal or vaginal area. The worms may be seen with a flashlight as 0.5" long crawling threads in the area of the anus after the child has been asleep for about an hour.
- See a health professional for treatment recommendations.
- Bathe the child in the morning to remove a large proportion of eggs that are laid at night.
- Frequently change underwear, bedclothes, and bedsheets to decrease egg contamination.
- Wash children's hands directly after using the toilet, and also before hands are involved with putting something into their mouths.
- Wash toys frequently.
- Clean and sanitize surfaces used for eating, toileting, hand washing, food preparation, and diapering.

Exclude from group setting?

No.

Comments

- Pinworms are not dangerous.
- Pinworms are relatively common among preschool- and school-aged children and easily shared within these groups.
- In the past, pinworms were found in 5% to 15% of the US population, but incidence has since decreased.

American Academy of Pediatrics

DEDICATED TO THE HEALTH OF ALL CHILDREN™

The American Academy of Pediatrics is an organization of 60,000 primary care pediatricians, pediatric medical subspecialists, and pediatric surgical specialists dedicated to the health, safety, and well-being of infants, children, adolescents, and young adults.

American Academy of Pediatrics
PO Box 747
Elk Grove Village, IL 60009-0747
Web site—http://www.aap.org

Pneumonia

What is pneumonia?

An inflammation of the lungs primarily caused by a viral or bacterial infection. Infection of the lungs often is secondary to an infection that starts in the nose and throat area (ie, the upper portion of the respiratory tract) and then spreads to the lungs (ie, the lower portion of the respiratory tract). The infection can start in the lungs from an infection brought there by the blood (especially pneumonia caused by bacterial infection).

What are the signs or symptoms?

- Cough
- Fast, difficult breathing
- Fever
- Muscle aches
- Loss of appetite
- Lethargy

What are the incubation and contagious periods?

- Incubation period: Pneumonia is a condition caused by a variety of types of germs (organisms); therefore, incubation periods will vary depending on the germ causing the pneumonia.
- Contagious period: Depends on the germ causing the pneumonia.

How is it spread?

Pneumonia does not spread. The germ that causes the pneumonia can spread if the person is still infectious at the time the pneumonia develops. Most of the germs that cause pneumonia spread by direct or close contact with mouth and nose secretions and touching contaminated objects.

How do you control it?

- Good hand washing techniques.
- Teach children and caregivers/teachers to cover their noses and mouths when sneezing or coughing with a disposable facial tissue if possible, or with a shoulder if no facial tissue is available in time ("give your cough or sneeze a cold shoulder"). Teach everyone to remove any soil, change or cover contaminated clothing, and wash their hands right after using facial tissues or having contact with mucus to prevent the spread of disease by contaminated hands.
- Dispose of facial tissues that contain nasal secretions after each use.
- Sanitize surfaces that are touched by hands frequently such as toys, tables, and doorknobs according to the schedule on page 14.

What are the roles of the caregiver/teacher and the family?

- Immunizations prevent some of the bacterial infections that cause pneumonia. Influenza vaccine may prevent pneumonia that sometimes occurs as a complication of influenza infection.
- Be sure children 6 to 23 months of age, children at high risk from influenza, and their caregivers/teachers receive influenza vaccine each fall. Influenza vaccine should be considered for all children in group care settings and their caregivers/teachers because they are at increased risk for influenza infection.

Exclude from group setting?

No, unless

- The child is unable to participate and staff determine that they cannot care for the child without compromising their ability to care for the health and safety of the other children in the group.
- The child meets other exclusion criteria, such as fever with behavior change (see "Conditions Requiring Temporary Exclusion" on page 28).

Readmit to group setting?

When exclusion criteria are resolved, the child is able to participate, and staff determine that they can care for the child without compromising their ability to care for the health and safety of the other children in the group

Comment

Because most forms of pneumonia are linked to viral or bacterial infections that spread from person to person, they are most common during the fall, winter, and early spring, when children spend more time indoors in close contact with others.

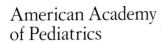

American Academy of Pediatrics

DEDICATED TO THE HEALTH OF ALL CHILDREN™

The American Academy of Pediatrics is an organization of 60,000 primary care pediatricians, pediatric medical subspecialists, and pediatric surgical specialists dedicated to the health, safety, and well-being of infants, children, adolescents, and young adults.

American Academy of Pediatrics
PO Box 747
Elk Grove Village, IL 60009-0747
Web site—http://www.aap.org

Respiratory Syncytial Virus (RSV)

What is respiratory syncytial virus?

- A virus that causes the common cold and other respiratory signs or symptoms
- Most common in winter and early spring, but can occur year-round

What are the signs or symptoms?

- Cold-like signs or symptoms for most children.
- Very young infants exhibit
  - ~ Irritability.
  - ~ Poor feeding.
  - ~ Lethargy.
  - ~ Cyanosis (ie, turn blue with cough or brief periods of no breathing).
- Respiratory problems include
  - ~ Bronchiolitis (ie, wheezing from narrowed airways in the lungs).
  - ~ Pneumonia.
- Children with weakened immune systems, prematurity, or heart or lung problems have greater difficulty when ill with this infection.

What are the incubation and contagious periods?

- Incubation period: 2 to 8 days; 4 to 6 days is most common.
- Contagious period: The virus can be shed for 3 to 8 days (3 to 4 weeks in young infants, usually beginning a day or so before signs or symptoms appear).

How is it spread?

- Direct or close contact with mouth or nose secretions.
- The virus can live on surfaces for many hours and 30 minutes or more on hands.
- Before signs or symptoms appear, the infected person starts to shed virus that may infect others.

How do you control it?

- Hand washing.
- Prevent contact with respiratory secretions. Teach children and caregivers/teachers to cover their noses and mouths when sneezing or coughing with a disposable facial tissue if possible, or with a shoulder if no facial tissue is available in time ("give your cough or sneeze a cold shoulder"). Teach everyone to remove any soil, change or cover contaminated clothing, and wash their hands right after using facial tissues or having contact with mucus to prevent the spread of disease by contaminated hands.

- Dispose of used facial tissues that contain nasal secretions after each use.
- Although separation of ill children and use of gowns and masks is not practical in child care and school settings, based on studies of control of this infection in hospital settings, several measures may be considered.
  - ~ Make sure that hand washing facilities are close at hand to encourage hand hygiene (see "Hand Washing Steps" on page 17), especially before and after any activity involving food or touching the mouth, nose, and eyes.
  - ~ Sanitize commonly touched surfaces more frequently during the winter and early spring when outbreaks can be expected.
  - ~ Caregivers/teachers who are likely to get nasal secretions on their clothing through close contact with children may help reduce the spread by keeping a spare shirt or smock handy to change into if their clothing becomes contaminated.

What are the roles of the caregiver/teacher and the family?

- Report the infection to staff designated by the child care program or school for decision making and action related to care of ill children. That person, in turn, alerts possibly exposed family members and staff to watch for symptoms.
- Practice control measures at home and in group care settings.

Exclude from group setting?

No, unless

- Child exhibits rapid or labored breathing or cyanotic (blue) episodes.
- The child is unable to participate and staff determine that they cannot care for the child without compromising their ability to care for the health and safety of the other children in the group.
- The child meets other exclusion criteria, such as fever with behavior change (see "Conditions Requiring Temporary Exclusion" on page 28).

Readmit to group setting?

When exclusion criteria are resolved, the child is able to participate, and staff determine that they can care for the child without compromising their ability to care for the health and safety of the other children in the group

➤ continued

Respiratory Syncytial Virus (RSV), continued

Comments

- Almost all children are infected at least once by 2 years of age, and reinfection during life is common.
- Certain infants and young children at high risk (eg, extreme prematurity, heart or lung problems) may benefit from a monthly injection of an antibody to RSV at the beginning of and continuing throughout the RSV season.
- All children should be protected from exposure to tobacco smoke, and special efforts to avoid tobacco smoke are warranted for children who are at risk for serious disease from RSV.

American Academy
of Pediatrics

DEDICATED TO THE HEALTH OF ALL CHILDREN™

The American Academy of Pediatrics is an organization of 60,000 primary care pediatricians, pediatric medical subspecialists, and pediatric surgical specialists dedicated to the health, safety, and well-being of infants, children, adolescents, and young adults.

American Academy of Pediatrics
PO Box 747
Elk Grove Village, IL 60009-0747
Web site—http://www.aap.org

Ringworm (Tinea)

What is ringworm?

A fungal infection that may affect the body, feet, or scalp

What are the signs or symptoms?

- Skin
  - ~ Red, circular patches with raised edges and central clearing
  - ~ Cracking and peeling of skin between toes
- Scalp
  - ~ Patchy areas of dandruff-like scaling with or without hair loss
  - ~ Redness and scaling of scalp with broken hairs or patches of hair loss

What are the incubation and contagious periods?

Unknown

How is it spread?

- Direct person-to-person contact by sharing combs, brushes, towels, clothing, or bedding
- Fungus infection spread by contact with infected humans, animals (eg, cats, dogs), or contaminated surfaces or objects
- Mildly infectious as long as the lesions are not treated

How do you control it?

- Early treatment of infected people.
- Examination of siblings and other household contacts.
- Do not share ribbons, combs, or hairbrushes.
- Cover skin lesions.

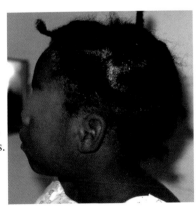

Child with ringworm of the scalp

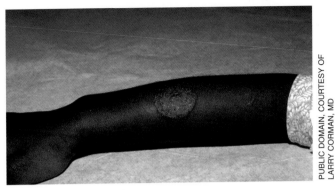

PUBLIC DOMAIN, COURTESY OF LARRY CORMAN, MD

Child with ringworm of the forearm

What are the roles of the caregiver/teacher and the family?

- Report the infection to staff designated by the child care program or school for decision making and action related to care of ill children. That person, in turn, alerts possibly exposed family members and staff to watch for symptoms.
- Give medication as prescribed.
- On arrival and by observation while the child is in care, note any areas of the skin or scalp that might be infected.
- Do not permit the sharing of bike helmets, hats, combs, brushes, barrettes, scarves, clothing, bedding, or towels.
- Restructure dress-up corner by laundering an outfit before a second child wears it or having disposable outfits.

Exclude from group setting?

Yes, at the end of the program or school day.

Readmit to group setting?

Once treatment is started.

Comments

- Extreme measures of shaving head or wearing a cap are unnecessary.
- Ringworm of the scalp occurs most commonly in children between 3 and 9 years of age and seems to be more common in African American children.

PAUL HONIG, MD

American Academy of Pediatrics

DEDICATED TO THE HEALTH OF ALL CHILDREN™

The American Academy of Pediatrics is an organization of 60,000 primary care pediatricians, pediatric medical subspecialists, and pediatric surgical specialists dedicated to the health, safety, and well-being of infants, children, adolescents, and young adults.

American Academy of Pediatrics
PO Box 747
Elk Grove Village, IL 60009-0747
Web site—http://www.aap.org

Roseola (Human Herpesvirus 6)

What is roseola?

A viral infection causing rash in infants and children that primarily occurs between 6 and 24 months of age

What are the signs or symptoms?

- High fever (above 103°F) lasting 3 to 7 days.
  - ~ Fever may cause seizure activity.
  - ~ Often, the child is not very ill when fever is present.
- Red, raised rash lasting from hours to several days that becomes apparent the day the fever breaks (usually the fourth day).

What are the incubation and contagious periods?

- Incubation period: 9 to 10 days
- Contagious period: Unknown

How is it spread?

- Person-to-person contact.
- Virus sometimes exists in nose or throat excretions of healthy people who have had the disease in the past.
- Nearly all individuals get this infection early in life, some without signs or symptoms. Most children have had the infection by the time they are 4 years of age.
- Most likely source of transmission to children is healthy adults. Saliva from three fourths of adults without symptoms contains infectious virus.

How do you control it?

Hand washing

What are the roles of the caregiver/teacher and the family?

- Report the infection to staff designated by the child care program or school for decision making and action related to care of ill children. That person, in turn, alerts possibly exposed family members and staff to watch for symptoms.
- Inform parents about the nature of the illness and that while the fever phase of the illness can cause concern, once the rash appears, the child is in the recovery phase.

Exclude from group setting?

No, unless

- The child is unable to participate and staff determine that they cannot care for the child without compromising their ability to care for the health and safety of the other children in the group.
- The child meets other exclusion criteria, such as fever with behavior change (see "Conditions Requiring Temporary Exclusion" on page 28).

Readmit to group setting?

When exclusion criteria are resolved, the child is able to participate, and staff determine that they can care for the child without compromising their ability to care for the health and safety of the other children in the group

American Academy of Pediatrics

DEDICATED TO THE HEALTH OF ALL CHILDREN™

The American Academy of Pediatrics is an organization of 60,000 primary care pediatricians, pediatric medical subspecialists, and pediatric surgical specialists dedicated to the health, safety, and well-being of infants, children, adolescents, and young adults.

American Academy of Pediatrics
PO Box 747
Elk Grove Village, IL 60009-0747
Web site—http://www.aap.org

Rotavirus

What is rotavirus?

- A virus that belongs to a family of viruses found worldwide as one of the most common causes of diarrhea and vomiting.
- The single most common cause of diarrhea in children younger than 2 years.
- Disease occurs more frequently in cooler months (ie, late autumn to early spring).
- Nearly all children have been infected by the time they reach 3 years of age.
- Children can get infected more than once because the virus has many types.

What are the signs or symptoms?

- Non-bloody diarrhea
- Nausea
- Vomiting
- Dehydration in severe cases
- Generally lasts 3 to 8 days

What are the incubation and contagious periods?

- Incubation period: 2 to 4 days.
- Contagious period: Virus is present before diarrhea begins and can persist for up to 3 weeks after the illness.

How is it spread?

- Fecal-oral route (Organism can be found on toys and hard surfaces.)
- Often spread within families

How do you control it?

- Hand washing, especially after toileting or diapering and before any contact with food or surfaces involved in preparation and serving food.
- Surface sanitation that includes cleaning and rinsing of surfaces with detergent and water and then application of a 70% ethanol solution that is allowed to air-dry or a sprayed on, freshly made 1:64 dilution of household bleach (1 tablespoon of household bleach to 1 quart of water) that completely wets the surface for at least 2 minutes.
- Two rotavirus vaccines are currently under investigation.

What are the roles of the caregiver/teacher and the family?

- Report the infection to staff designated by the child care program or school for decision making and action related to care of ill children. That person, in turn, alerts possibly exposed family members and staff to watch for symptoms.
- During outbreaks, reeducate staff to ensure strict and frequent hand washing, diapering, toileting, food handling and cleaning, and sanitation procedures.

Exclude from group setting?

Yes, if

- The child has diarrhea not contained in the toilet (all infants and children who use diapers or have toileting accidents and have diarrhea must be excluded).
- Child has diarrhea and is able to use the toilet, but he or she has no urine output in 8 hours (suggesting that the child's diarrhea may be associated with dehydration).
- The child is unable to participate and staff determine that they cannot care for the child without compromising their ability to care for the health and safety of the other children in the group.
- The child meets other exclusion criteria, such as fever with behavior change (see "Conditions Requiring Temporary Exclusion" on page 28).

Readmit to group setting?

- Stool is contained in toilet (for toilet-trained children).
- Even if stools stay loose, if the child seems well and the stool consistency has not changed for a week.
- When the child is able to participate and staff determine that they can care for the child without compromising their ability to care for the health and safety of the other children in the group.

American Academy
of Pediatrics

DEDICATED TO THE HEALTH OF ALL CHILDREN™

The American Academy of Pediatrics is an organization of 60,000 primary care pediatricians, pediatric medical subspecialists, and pediatric surgical specialists dedicated to the health, safety, and well-being of infants, children, adolescents, and young adults.

American Academy of Pediatrics
PO Box 747
Elk Grove Village, IL 60009-0747
Web site—http://www.aap.org

Rubella (German Measles)

What is rubella?

A mild viral infection usually lasting 3 days that is now rare in the United States because of routine immunization

What are the signs or symptoms?

- Many children have no signs or symptoms.
- Red or pink rash appearing first on the face, then spreading downward over the body.
- Swollen glands behind ears.
- Slight fever.
- May experience joint aches and/or pain (rare in children; more common in adults).

What are the incubation and contagious periods?

- Incubation period: 14 to 23 days; usually 16 to 18 days
- Contagious period: May be spread 7 days before to 14 days after the rash

How is it spread?

- Respiratory route (droplets from sneezing or coughing)
- Direct contact with nose or throat secretions

How do you control it?

- Immunize according to the current recommendations.
- Review immunization status of all children.
- Unimmunized children should be excluded from group care settings if there is an outbreak.

What are the roles of the caregiver/teacher and the family?

- Report the infection to staff designated by the child care program or school for decision making and action related to care of ill children. That person, in turn, alerts possibly exposed family members and staff to watch for symptoms.
- Report the infection to the health department, as the health professional who makes the diagnosis may not report that the child who has the infection is a participant in a child care program or school, and this could lead to precious time for controlling the spread of the disease being lost.
- Staff who care for children should have immunity documented because rubella infection during pregnancy can result in miscarriage, fetal death, or severe abnormalities in the formation and function of organ systems in the fetus, including mental retardation.

Exclude from group setting?

Yes.

- Rubella is a highly communicable illness for which routine exclusion of infected children is warranted.
- For outbreaks, exclude exposed children who have not been immunized until they become immunized or, if they are not immunized because of an accepted exemption, continue to exclude them until the health department determines it is safe for them to return.

Readmit to group setting?

- Six days after onset of rash
- When the child is able to participate and staff determine that they can care for the child without compromising their ability to care for the health and safety of the other children in the group

American Academy
of Pediatrics

DEDICATED TO THE HEALTH OF ALL CHILDREN™

The American Academy of Pediatrics is an organization of 60,000 primary care pediatricians, pediatric medical subspecialists, and pediatric surgical specialists dedicated to the health, safety, and well-being of infants, children, adolescents, and young adults.

American Academy of Pediatrics
PO Box 747
Elk Grove Village, IL 60009-0747
Web site—http://www.aap.org

Salmonella

What is *Salmonella?*

An intestinal infection caused by *Salmonella* bacteria

What are the signs or symptoms?

- Diarrhea
- Fever
- Abdominal cramps and tenderness
- Nausea or vomiting
- Sometimes blood or mucus in stool

What are the incubation and contagious periods?

- Incubation period: 6 to 48 hours.
- Contagious period: Half of children still have *Salmonella* in stool 12 weeks after infection.

How is it spread?

- Fecal-oral route from infected people and animals, especially from reptiles and poultry
- Ingestion of contaminated food, water, meats, eggs, and unpasteurized milk
- Direct contact with infected objects or surfaces

How do you control it?

- Hand washing.
- No reptiles (eg, turtles, salamanders, snakes) as pets for children. *Salmonella* is a normal bacterial inhabitant of the intestinal tract of reptiles. Cages and all surfaces involved in the care of reptiles should be considered likely to be contaminated with this organism and a source that spreads infection to children in group care settings.
- Proper sanitation methods for food processing, preparation, and service. Special attention is necessary to avoid contamination by raw poultry or surfaces such as cutting boards and utensils.
- Eggs and other foods of animal origin should be cooked thoroughly.

What are the roles of the caregiver/teacher and the family?

- Report the infection to staff designated by the child care program or school for decision making and action related to care of ill children. That person, in turn, alerts possibly exposed family members and staff to watch for symptoms.
- Report the infection to the health department, as the health professional who makes the diagnosis may not report that the child who has the infection is a participant in a child care program or school, and this could lead to precious time for controlling the spread of the disease being lost.
- Infected people should not be involved in food preparation.
- Prevent contact of young children with reptiles and poultry. Ensure immediate hand washing if there has been any contact with these animals.

Exclude from group setting?

Yes, if

- Child has diarrhea not contained in the toilet (all infants and children in diapers who have diarrhea must be excluded).
- For children who have diarrhea and are able to use the toilet, exclude if the child has had no urine output in 8 hours (suggesting that the child's diarrhea may be causing dehydration).
- The child is unable to participate and staff determine that they cannot care for the child without compromising their ability to care for the health and safety of the other children in the group.
- The child meets other exclusion criteria, such as fever with behavior change (see "Conditions Requiring Temporary Exclusion" on page 28).

Readmit to group setting?

- Health professional must clear child for readmission for all cases of *Salmonella.*
- Three negative test results from stool cultures are needed for children with *Salmonella typhi,* but other types of *Salmonella* do not require negative test results from stool cultures.
- Stool is contained in the toilet (for toilet-trained children).
- Even if stools stay loose, if the child seems well and the stool consistency has not changed for a week.

➤ *continued*

Salmonella, continued

- When the child is able to participate and staff determine that they can care for the child without compromising their ability to care for the health and safety of the other children in the group.

Comments

- Outbreaks in group care settings are rare.
- Antibiotics usually are not indicated.
- Age-specific attack rates are highest in children younger than 4 years.

American Academy
of Pediatrics

DEDICATED TO THE HEALTH OF ALL CHILDREN™

The American Academy of Pediatrics is an organization of 60,000 primary care pediatricians, pediatric medical subspecialists, and pediatric surgical specialists dedicated to the health, safety, and well-being of infants, children, adolescents, and young adults.

American Academy of Pediatrics
PO Box 747
Elk Grove Village, IL 60009-0747
Web site—http://www.aap.org

Scabies

What is scabies?

An infestation of the skin by small insects called mites

What are the signs or symptoms?

- Rash, severe itching (increased at night).
- Itchy red bumps or blisters found on skin folds between the fingers, toes, wrists, elbows, armpits, waistline, thighs, penis, abdomen, and lower buttocks.
- Children younger than 2 years are likely to be infested on the head, neck, palms, and soles of feet or in a diffuse distribution over the body.

What are the incubation and contagious periods?

- Incubation period
  ~ Four to 6 weeks for those who have never been infected.
  ~ One to 4 days for those who have been previously infected (repeated exposures tend to be milder).
- Contagious period: Until the insect infestation is treated.

How is it spread?

- Person-to-person contact
- Sharing of bedding, towels, and clothing

How do you control it?

- Launder bedding and clothing (hot water and hot drying cycle) worn next to skin at least 4 days before start of treatment.
- Items that cannot be laundered should be placed in plastic bags for at least 4 days.

What are the roles of the caregiver/teacher and the family?

- Report the infection to staff designated by the child care program or school for decision making and action related to care of ill children. That person, in turn, alerts possibly exposed family members and staff to watch for symptoms.
- Contact health professional if itching continues after several weeks of treatment.
- Family members and very close contacts should be treated at the same time as the child, even if no signs or symptoms are present.

Exclude from group setting?

Yes, until after treatment is completed.

Readmit to group setting?

After treatment has been completed (usually overnight)

Comment

Scabies affects people from all socioeconomic levels without regard to sex, age, or personal hygiene.

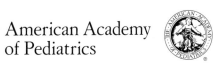

American Academy
of Pediatrics

DEDICATED TO THE HEALTH OF ALL CHILDREN™

The American Academy of Pediatrics is an organization of 60,000 primary care pediatricians, pediatric medical subspecialists, and pediatric surgical specialists dedicated to the health, safety, and well-being of infants, children, adolescents, and young adults.

American Academy of Pediatrics
PO Box 747
Elk Grove Village, IL 60009-0747
Web site—http://www.aap.org

Shigella

What is *Shigella*?

An infection caused by the *Shigella* bacteria.

What are the signs or symptoms?

- Loose, watery stools with blood or mucus
- Fever
- Headache
- Convulsions
- Abdominal pain

What are the incubation and contagious periods?

- Incubation period: 1 to 7 days; average is 2 to 4 days.
- Contagious period: Untreated, *Shigella* persists in stool for up to 4 weeks.

How is it spread?

- Fecal-oral route.
- Very small numbers of organisms can cause infection.
- Children 5 years or younger, adults who care for young children, and others living in crowded conditions are at increased risk of outbreaks.

How do you control it?

- Hand washing.
- Eliminate access to shared water play areas.
- Adherence to sanitary diaper changing techniques.
- Sanitary food handling, including measures to decrease contamination of food by houseflies and assurance that any staff with diarrhea are not involved in food handling or feeding.
- Culture stool from other people with diarrhea when a child or staff member is diagnosed with *Shigella* so that all those whose culture results are positive are treated with antibiotics and excluded until diarrhea stops and test results from stool cultures are negative for *Shigella*. If several people are infected, they may be grouped together (as a cohort) until their test results from stool cultures are negative for *Shigella*.
- Note: While most infections are self-limited, antibiotics are effective in shortening the duration of diarrhea and eliminating the *Shigella* bacteria.

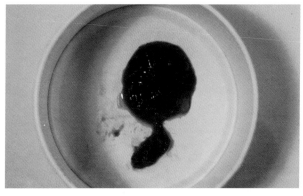

Bloody stool from a child with *Shigella* infection

What are the roles of the caregiver/teacher and the family?

- Report the infection to staff designated by the child care program or school for decision making and action related to care of ill children. That person, in turn, alerts possibly exposed family members and staff to watch for symptoms.
- Report the infection to the health department, as the health professional who makes the diagnosis may not report that the child who has the infection is a participant in a child care program or school, and this could lead to precious time for controlling the spread of the disease being lost.
- Stop food handling or feeding of others by individuals with diarrhea.

Exclude from group setting?

Yes. Exclude infected individuals until treatment is complete and test results from stool cultures are negative.

Readmit to group setting?

- When infected individuals are treated and test results from 2 stool cultures taken 24 hours apart are negative.
- Health professional must clear child for readmission for all cases of *Shigella*.
- Stool is contained in toilet (for toilet-trained children).
- Diarrhea is resolved for diapered children.
- When the child is able to participate and staff determine that they can care for the child without compromising their ability to care for the health and safety of the other children in the group.

American Academy of Pediatrics

DEDICATED TO THE HEALTH OF ALL CHILDREN™

The American Academy of Pediatrics is an organization of 60,000 primary care pediatricians, pediatric medical subspecialists, and pediatric surgical specialists dedicated to the health, safety, and well-being of infants, children, adolescents, and young adults.

American Academy of Pediatrics
PO Box 747
Elk Grove Village, IL 60009-0747
Web site — http://www.aap.org

Shingles (Herpes Zoster)

What is shingles?

An infection caused by the reactivation of varicella-zoster (chickenpox) virus within the body of someone who previously had chickenpox or (rarely) someone who had received the chickenpox vaccine in the past

What are the signs or symptoms?

Appearance of red bumps and blisters, usually in a narrow area on half of the body, that may be itchy or painful.

What are the incubation and contagious periods?

- Incubation period: The virus can remain in the body in an inactive state for many years after the first infection as chickenpox. Shingles may occur many years after having chickenpox when the virus (varicella-zoster) reactivates.
- Contagious period: Until the blisters are covered by scabs.

How is it spread?

Direct contact with blisters

How do you control it?

- Careful hand washing technique
- Covering blisters

What are the roles of the caregiver/teacher and the family?

- Report the infection to staff designated by the child care program or school for decision making and action related to care of ill children. That person, in turn, alerts possibly exposed family members and staff to watch for symptoms.
- Inform others of the greater risk to
  ~ Susceptible adults and children
  ~ Children or adults with impaired immune systems

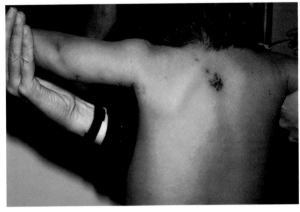

Child with shingles

PAUL HONIG, MD

Exclude from group setting?

No, unless

- The rash cannot be covered.
- The child is unable to participate and staff determine that they cannot care for the child without compromising their ability to care for the health and safety of the other children in the group.
- The child meets other exclusion criteria, such as fever with behavior change (see "Conditions Requiring Temporary Exclusion" on page 28).

Readmit to group setting?

- When rash can be covered or when all lesions have crusted
- When the child is able to participate and staff determine that they can care for the child without compromising their ability to care for the health and safety of the other children in the group

Comment

The virus that causes shingles is the virus that causes chickenpox. Vaccination of susceptible individuals is the best way to prevent or decrease the severity of infection with this virus.

American Academy of Pediatrics

DEDICATED TO THE HEALTH OF ALL CHILDREN™

The American Academy of Pediatrics is an organization of 60,000 primary care pediatricians, pediatric medical subspecialists, and pediatric surgical specialists dedicated to the health, safety, and well-being of infants, children, adolescents, and young adults.

American Academy of Pediatrics
PO Box 747
Elk Grove Village, IL 60009-0747
Web site—http://www.aap.org

Strep Throat (Streptococcal Pharyngitis) and Scarlet Fever

What is strep throat?

A disease caused by group A streptococcus bacteria

What is scarlet fever?

- Strep throat accompanied by a fine red rash that makes the skin feel like very fine sandpaper. The rash is usually more prominent in the armpits and groin area, often making the creases in the bend of the elbow and back of the knee pinker than usual. Sometimes the area around the mouth has a pale appearance compared with adjacent skin.
- The presence of the rash does not increase the severity of the disease.

What are the signs or symptoms?

- Some of the following may be present:
  ~ Sore throat
  ~ Fever
  ~ Stomachache
  ~ Headache
  ~ Swollen lymph nodes in neck
  ~ Decreased appetite
- Strep throat is much less likely if there is
  ~ Runny nose
  ~ Cough
  ~ Congestion
- Children younger than 3 years with group A streptococcal infection rarely have a sore throat. Most commonly, these children have a persistent nasal discharge (which may be associated with a foul odor from the mouth), fever, irritability, and loss of appetite.

What are the incubation and contagious periods?

- Incubation period: 2 to 5 days.
- Contagious period: The risk of spread is reduced when a person who is ill with strep throat is treated with antibiotics, but many people carry the bacteria that cause strep throat in their nose and throat and are not ill. In outbreaks in child care settings and schools, throat cultures of children who have no signs or symptoms have yielded positive test results in 15% to 50% of those tested. The percentage of carriage during times other than outbreaks is much less (5% to 10%). The risk of transmission from someone who is not sick but is carrying the bacteria is minimal. Note that the bacteria that cause strep throat also can cause impetigo.

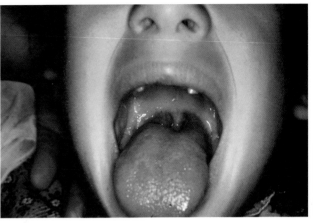

NEAL HALSEY, MD

Child with strep throat

How is it spread?

- Direct contact.
- Respiratory droplets.
- Close contact helps the spread of the infection.

How do you control it?

- Hand washing.
- Have a health professional evaluate individuals with a severe sore throat with a rash or severe sore throat that lasts more than 24 hours and is not associated with other signs or symptoms of a cold so that the person can be tested to determine if the cause is strep throat.

What are the roles of the caregiver/teacher and the family?

- Report the infection to staff designated by the child care program or school for decision making and action related to care of ill children. That person, in turn, alerts possibly exposed family members and staff to watch for symptoms.
- Antibiotics for infected individuals.

Exclude from group setting?
Yes.

Readmit to group setting?

- After 24 hours of antibiotic treatment
- When the child is able to participate and staff determine that they can care for the child without compromising their ability to care for the health and safety of the other children in the group

➤ *continued*

Strep Throat (Streptococcal Pharyngitis) and Scarlet Fever, continued

Comments

- Children usually do not pass the streptococcal bacteria to others once they have been on an antibiotic for 24 hours.
- Most frequent cause of sore throat in children is viral infection, not strep throat.
- A throat culture or rapid strep test is the only way to be certain of the diagnosis of strep throat.
- Even if untreated, most children and adults with group A streptococcal infections recover on their own. Some who are not treated develop complications including ear infections, sinusitis, abscesses in the tonsils, or infection of the lymph nodes (ie, tender and warm "swollen glands"). Indications for testing include a sudden development of sore throat, fever, headache, pain on swallowing, abdominal pain, nausea, vomiting, and enlarged tender lymph nodes in the front part of the neck.

- The concern about this infection is related to complications involving the heart and kidneys that can follow group A streptococcal infection. Children younger than 3 years who have this infection may have a runny nose and then get fever and other signs of illness. Children of this younger age group are very unlikely to suffer from rheumatic heart disease—the primary reason for treatment. However, outbreaks of strep throat have been reported in young children in group care settings. Testing for strep in these young children may be indicated when they are in contact with older children and caregivers/teachers in a group care setting, but would not be indicated otherwise.

American Academy of Pediatrics

DEDICATED TO THE HEALTH OF ALL CHILDREN™

The American Academy of Pediatrics is an organization of 60,000 primary care pediatricians, pediatric medical subspecialists, and pediatric surgical specialists dedicated to the health, safety, and well-being of infants, children, adolescents, and young adults.

American Academy of Pediatrics
PO Box 747
Elk Grove Village, IL 60009-0747
Web site—http://www.aap.org

Tuberculosis (TB)

What is tuberculosis?

An infection caused by the bacterium *Mycobacterium tuberculosis* that usually involves the lungs, but could affect other parts of the body

What are the signs or symptoms?

- Most TB infections in children and adolescents are without signs or symptoms.
- When infection causes disease, signs or symptoms most often occur 1 to 6 months after infection occurs and include
  ~ Chronic cough
  ~ Weight loss
  ~ Fever
  ~ Growth delay
  ~ Night sweats
  ~ Chills
- Infection is most often diagnosed by a positive TB skin test result. A chest x-ray film is needed for those with a positive skin test to determine the extent of the infection and the necessary treatment.

What are the incubation and contagious periods?

- Incubation period: The bacteria can be carried in the body for many years without active disease.
- Contagious period: Generally, infants and young children with active TB disease are not contagious. This is because they do not form cavities in their lungs with secretions that contain the TB bacterium, and when they cough, they do not create enough force to expel large numbers of TB germs into the air. Adolescents and adults who have active TB spread the disease by coughing and contaminating the environment as long as the disease is active.

How is it spread?

- Infection in children is nearly always the result of close contact with an adult who has TB.
- Respiratory route through coughing or sneezing, usually in an indoor environment.
- People are only contagious when there is active disease in their lungs or throat that has not been treated.
- It is *not* spread through clothes, dishes, floors, or furniture.

How do you control it?

- Require regular and substitute staff and volunteers to have a 1- or 2-step Mantoux intradermal skin test prior to employment. A 1-step test involves having the skin test only once. A 2-step test requires having 2 tests, usually about a month apart, to "boost" the response of the person. The 2-step test is used for people who are suspected to have a weakened immune system.
- In some cases, skin testing of children and staff may be necessary if exposed to TB.
- Exclusion and treatment of caregivers/teachers with active disease; skin testing of all contacts of adults with active disease.

What are the roles of the caregiver/teacher and the family?

- Report the infection to staff designated by the child care program or school for decision making and action related to care of ill children. That person, in turn, alerts possibly exposed family members and staff to watch for symptoms.
- Immediate notification of local and/or state health authorities of suspected cases involving children or staff.
- Ensure that children and staff take all prescribed medication. Directly observed treatment is essential.
- Staff with previously positive skin test results should be evaluated by their health professionals anytime they develop a disease that involves fever, night sweats, weight loss, or persistent coughing to assess their need for treatment and any risk of contagion related to their TB status.

Exclude from group setting?
Yes.

Readmit to group setting?

- As soon as effective therapy has been started and adherence to medication is documented
- When the child is approved to return by local health officials and considered noninfectious to others
- When the child is able to participate and staff determine that they can care for the child without compromising their ability to care for the health and safety of the other children in the group

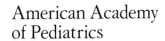

American Academy of Pediatrics

DEDICATED TO THE HEALTH OF ALL CHILDREN™

The American Academy of Pediatrics is an organization of 60,000 primary care pediatricians, pediatric medical subspecialists, and pediatric surgical specialists dedicated to the health, safety, and well-being of infants, children, adolescents, and young adults.

American Academy of Pediatrics
PO Box 747
Elk Grove Village, IL 60009-0747
Web site—http://www.aap.org

Upper Respiratory Infection (Common Cold)

What is an upper respiratory infection?

A viral infection of the upper respiratory tract (ie, nose, throat, ears, and eyes). Can also be a bacterial infection as in strep throat or sinusitis.

What are the signs or symptoms?

- Cough
- Sore or scratchy throat or tonsillitis
- Runny nose
- Sneezing or nasal discharge
- Watery eyes
- Headache
- Fever
- Earache

What are the incubation and contagious periods?

- Incubation period: 2 to 14 days.
- Contagious period: Usually a few days before signs or symptoms appear and while clear runny secretions are present. The presence of green or yellow discharge from the nose is common as the body discards mucus and other debris from the cold. These secretions do not contain a large load of virus and are less likely than the clear secretions to spread the cold virus to others.

How is it spread?

- Direct or close contact with mouth and nose secretions
- Touching contaminated objects

How do you control it?

- Good hand washing techniques.
- Teach children and caregivers/teachers to cover their noses and mouths when sneezing or coughing with a disposable facial tissue if possible, or with a shoulder if no facial tissue is available in time ("give your cough or sneeze a cold shoulder"). Teach everyone to remove any soil, change or cover contaminated clothing, and wash their hands right after using facial tissues or having contact with mucus to prevent the spread of disease by contaminated hands.
- Dispose of facial tissues that contain nasal secretions after each use.

- Sanitize surfaces that are touched by hands frequently, such as toys, tables, and doorknobs (see table on page 14).
- Ventilate the facility with fresh outdoor air and maintain temperature and humidity conditions as described in *Caring for Our Children,* Standard 5.028.
  - ~ Winter months: 65°F to 75°F with 30% to 50% relative humidity
  - ~ Summer months: 68°F to 82°F with 30% to 50% relative humidity
  - ~ Air exchange: Minimum of 15 cubic feet per minute per person of outdoor air

What are the roles of the caregiver/teacher and the family?

Exclusion of children with signs or symptoms has no benefit in reducing the spread of common respiratory infections. Viruses that cause upper respiratory infections are spread primarily by children who do not have signs or symptoms (ie, before they get sick, after they recover, often who never get sick).

Exclude from group setting?

No, unless

- The child is unable to participate and staff determine that they cannot care for the child without compromising their ability to care for the health and safety of the other children in the group.
- The child meets other exclusion criteria, such as fever with behavior change (see "Conditions Requiring Temporary Exclusion" on page 28).

Readmit to group setting?

When exclusion criteria are resolved, the child is able to participate, and staff determine that they can care for the child without compromising their ability to care for the health and safety of the other children in the group

➤ *continued*

Upper Respiratory Infection (Common Cold), continued

Comments

- Children in child care and school settings may have as many as 8 to 12 colds a year.
- As children get older, and the longer they are exposed to large numbers of children, they get fewer upper respiratory infections each year because of increased immunity. By 3 years of age, children who have been in group care since infancy have the same or fewer upper respiratory illnesses than children who are cared for only at home.

American Academy
of Pediatrics

DEDICATED TO THE HEALTH OF ALL CHILDREN™

The American Academy of Pediatrics is an organization of 60,000 primary care pediatricians, pediatric medical subspecialists, and pediatric surgical specialists dedicated to the health, safety, and well-being of infants, children, adolescents, and young adults.

American Academy of Pediatrics
PO Box 747
Elk Grove Village, IL 60009-0747
Web site—http://www.aap.org

Urinary Tract Infection

What is a urinary tract infection?

An infection of the urinary system, which includes the kidneys, the tubes that join the kidneys and bladder (ureters), the bladder, and the tube that leads from the bladder to the outside (the urethra). The most common urinary tract infections are caused by bacteria from feces on the skin that enter through the urethra to infect the bladder, particularly in girls. Anything that irritates the opening of the urethra can make it easier for infection to occur. In girls, the urethra is much shorter than in boys, so infection from the outside into the bladder happens more easily. Bathing in soapy water or a bubble bath can be irritating and predispose girls to getting urinary tract infections.

Some kidney infections occur by infection through the blood stream from an infection elsewhere in the body, especially in infants. This type of cause is uncommon. Most urinary tract infections occur from the spread of infection up the urinary tract from the outside.

What are the signs or symptoms?

- Pain when urinating
- Increased frequency of urinating
- Fever
- Loss of potty training after the child has had good control of urine for a period of time, especially when loss of control occurs in the daytime, with little warning

What are the incubation and contagious periods?

- Incubation period: Usually a few days.
- Contagious period: Urinary tract infections are not contagious.

How is it spread?

Irritation of the urinary tract

How do you control it?

- Dilute the urine by having the child drink fluids frequently. Diluting the urine gives bacteria less food to grow and makes it easier for the body to fight the infection.
- Have the child evaluated and treated by a health professional.
- Wipe the area around the genitalia from front to back, especially in girls, to avoid spreading fecal bacteria from the rectal into the urinary and vaginal area.

What are the roles of the caregiver/teacher and the family?

Exclusion of children with symptoms has no benefit in reducing the spread of urinary tract infections.

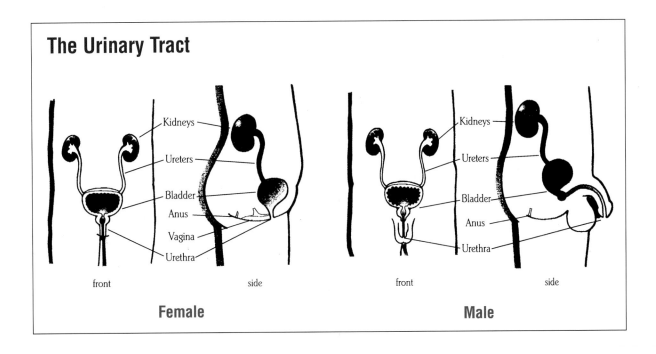

The Urinary Tract

Female — front — side

Male — front — side

Kidneys, Ureters, Bladder, Anus, Vagina, Urethra

Urinary Tract Infection, continued

Exclude from group setting?

No, unless

- The child is unable to participate and staff determine that they cannot care for the child without compromising their ability to care for the health and safety of the other children in the group.
- The child meets other exclusion criteria, such as fever with behavior change (see "Conditions Requiring Temporary Exclusion" on page 28).

Readmit to group setting?

When exclusion criteria are resolved, the child is able to participate, and staff determine that they can care for the child without compromising their ability to care for the health and safety of the other children in the group

Comment

A health professional should see a child with symptoms of a urinary tract infection for a diagnosis and proper treatment. Ignoring urinary tract symptoms can lead to damage to the kidneys, even if the symptoms seem to go away by themselves.

American Academy
of Pediatrics

DEDICATED TO THE HEALTH OF ALL CHILDREN™

The American Academy of Pediatrics is an organization of 60,000 primary care pediatricians, pediatric medical subspecialists, and pediatric surgical specialists dedicated to the health, safety, and well-being of infants, children, adolescents, and young adults.

American Academy of Pediatrics
PO Box 747
Elk Grove Village, IL 60009-0747
Web site—http://www.aap.org

Whooping Cough (Pertussis)

What is whooping cough?

A contagious and fairly common bacterial infection that causes a range of illnesses, from mild cough to severe disease

What are the signs or symptoms?

- Begins with cold-like signs or symptoms.
- Coughing that may progress to severe coughing which may cause
  ~ Vomiting.
  ~ Loss of breath, difficulty catching breath.
  ~ Cyanosis (ie, blueness).
- Whooping (ie, high-pitched crowing) sound when inhaling after a period of coughing (may not occur in very young children).
- Fever is usually absent or minimal.
- Symptoms more severe in children younger than 1 year.
- Infants may develop complications and often require hospitalization.

What are the incubation and contagious periods?

- Incubation period: 6 to 21 days; usually 7 to 10 days.
- Contagious period: From the beginning of symptoms until 2 weeks after the cough begins, depending on age, immunization status, previous episodes of infection with pertussis, and antibiotic treatment. An infant who has no pertussis immunizations may remain infectious for 6 weeks or more after the cough starts.

How is it spread?

- Direct or close contact with mouth and nose secretions
- Possibly by direct hand contact with contaminated secretions
- By children and adults who have a cough caused by pertussis, as in some cases of bronchitis

How do you control it?

- Whooping cough is a vaccine-preventable disease, although protection is incomplete and decreases over time after routine childhood immunization.
- Hand washing.

- Prophylactic antibiotics for household and other close contacts of an infected individual, including staff, and exposed, incompletely immunized children in group settings who have close or extensive contact with an individual with confirmed pertussis infection.
- Children who are incompletely immunized should complete their immunizations as well as receive the prophylactic antibiotic treatment.
- Test cultures of staff who develop respiratory symptoms after exposure to someone with confirmed pertussis.

What are the roles of the caregiver/teacher and the family?

- Report the infection to staff designated by the child care program or school for decision making and action related to care of ill children. That person, in turn, alerts possibly exposed family members and staff to watch for symptoms and seek prophylactic antibiotics.
- All adults who have contact with a child who has pertussis in group settings also should be advised to seek testing if symptoms develop.
- Report to local health authorities.
- Ensure that all children have received their immunization series according to the current recommendations.
- Monitor incompletely immunized children for respiratory signs or symptoms for 21 days after last contact with infected person.
- Monitor staff for respiratory signs or symptoms and recommend treatment if cough develops within 21 days of exposure.

Exclude from group setting?

Yes.
- Pertussis is a highly communicable illness for which routine exclusion of infected children is warranted.
- Exclude close contacts who are coughing until they receive appropriate evaluation and treatment.

Readmit to group setting?

- After 5 days of appropriate antibiotic treatment, which is given for a total of 14 days
- When the child is able to participate and staff determine that they can care for the child without compromising their ability to care for the health and safety of the other children in the group

American Academy
of Pediatrics

DEDICATED TO THE HEALTH OF ALL CHILDREN™

The American Academy of Pediatrics is an organization of 60,000 primary care pediatricians, pediatric medical subspecialists, and pediatric surgical specialists dedicated to the health, safety, and well-being of infants, children, adolescents, and young adults.

American Academy of Pediatrics
PO Box 747
Elk Grove Village, IL 60009-0747
Web site—http://www.aap.org

CHAPTER 8

Role of the Health Consultant in Child Care and Schools

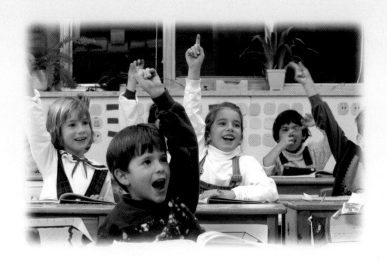

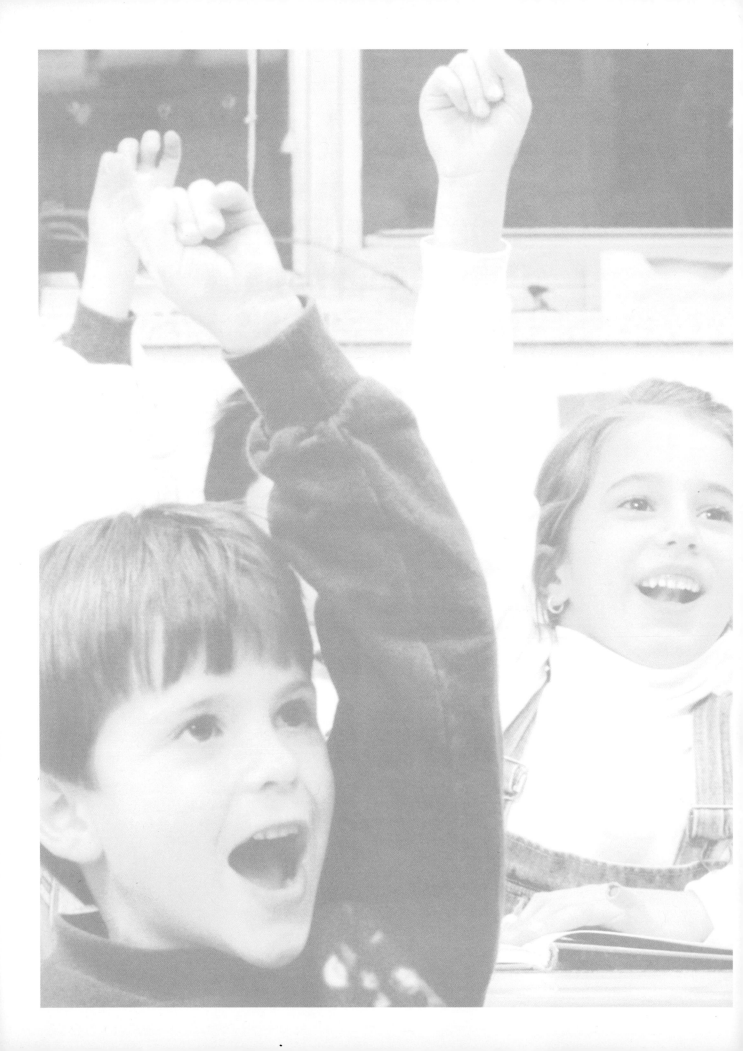

Role of the Health Consultant in Child Care and Schools

All child care and school settings should have access to a health consultant who can provide consultation and technical assistance. The health consultant is a health professional with expertise in child health and development who works with caregivers/teachers to recognize and promote the health and safety of staff, children, and families.

Who Is the Health Consultant?

The health consultant should be a pediatrician, family health physician, pediatric nurse practitioner, pediatric/community health nurse, or health professional with expertise in
- Mental health
- Nutrition
- Health education
- Oral health
- Environmental health
- Emergency management
- Infectious diseases
- Issues relating to caring for children with special health care needs

Although some state regulations require a health consultant, others do not. Please refer to the National Resource Center for Health and Safety in Child Care Web site (nrc.uchsc.edu) for the regulations for each state.

What Are the Qualifications of a Health Consultant?

The health consultant should have knowledge and expertise in the following areas:
- Routines, conditions, and constraints for caregivers/teachers
- Pediatric health care and early brain development
- Community, state, and national resources and regulations
- Principles of consultation
- Working with diverse populations
- Oral, written, and electronic communication
- Communication with non–health-related personnel and local health authorities
- Techniques to teach health and safety to adult learners who are not health professionals

What Does a Health Consultant Do?

The health consultant should be in regular contact with the child care program or school and able to
- Perform an assessment of the program focusing on health, safety, nutrition practices, and facility issues.
- Assist in the development and implementation of written health policies.
- Assist in linking children, families, and caregivers/teachers to community health resources including a medical home, immunizations, and health screenings.
- Contribute to the professional development of caregivers/teachers.
- Assist caregivers/teachers with the inclusion of children with special health care needs.
- Create health care plans for children with special health care needs, in collaboration with health professionals in the child's medical home.
- Delegate prescribed care to caregivers/teachers.
- Assist the program in the event of a communicable disease outbreak.

Why Does a Child Care Program or School Need a Health Consultant?

To assist in
- Preventing infectious diseases in children, staff, and families
- Preventing injuries
- Promoting health by using
  ~ Written policies
  ~ Food safety practices
  ~ Sanitation procedures
  ~ Play equipment assessments
  ~ Health record reviews
  ~ Illness and injury records
  ~ Education of staff and families

Where Can a Child Care Program or School Find a Health Consultant?

- Local health agencies.
- Local health clinics.
- Pediatric hospitals.
- Clinicians who care for children.
- State chapter of the American Academy of Pediatrics (www.aap.org).
- A parent who is a health professional (with appropriate limitations of access to confidential information about children and families in the program).
- Through the Healthy Child Care America program at www.healthychildcare.org.
- For more information about training of health consultants, visit the National Training Institute for Child Care Health Consultants Web site at www.sph.unc.edu/courses/childcare.

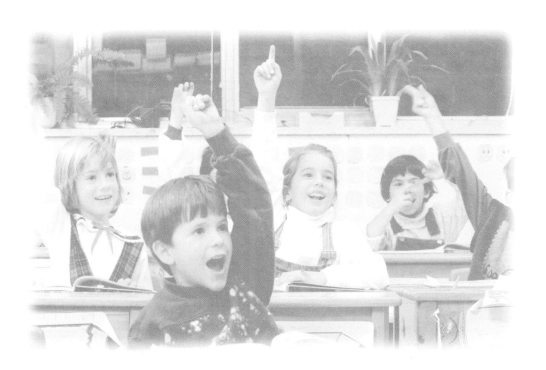

CHAPTER 9

Immunization Schedule and Information

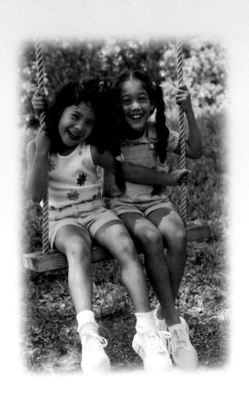

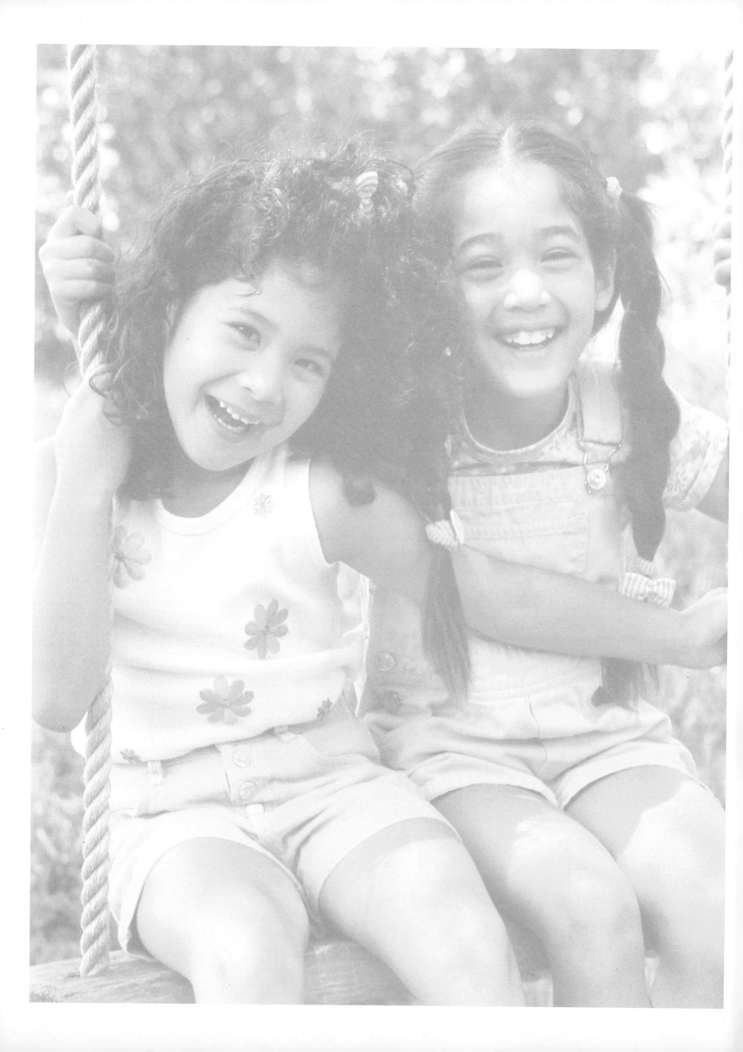

Immunization Schedule and Information

Preventing Diseases Through Routine Childhood Immunizations

Routine age-appropriate immunizations are the best means of preventing a large number of harmful childhood diseases. State laws requiring immunizations of children participating in group settings vary. Parents of all children should be encouraged to comply with the *Recommended Childhood and Adolescent Immunization Schedule* published on a regular basis, typically in January, by the Advisory Committee on Immunization Practices, American Academy of Pediatrics, and American Academy of Family Physicians (available online at www.cispimmunize.org and www.aapredbook.org). This schedule should be evaluated closely each year because it may include new vaccine products, timing, and number of injections. If there is a medical reason for not administering immunizations, a health professional's statement needs to be provided to the child care program or school with the reason why the child is exempt.

Unimmunized/Under-Immunized Children

Children who have not received all of their immunizations
- Should be immunized as soon as possible
- Should be allowed to attend group care unless one of the following vaccine-preventable disease to which they might be susceptible occurs in the program:
  ~ Diphtheria
  ~ *Haemophilus influenzae* type b
  ~ Hepatitis A virus (not routinely recommended in all states, but indicated in an outbreak if child is older than 2 years)
  ~ Influenza for 6- to 24-month-old children (Should be considered for all children in group care settings— see "Pneumonia" on page 101.)
  ~ Measles
  ~ Mumps
  ~ Pertussis
  ~ Polio
  ~ Rubella
  ~ Varicella
- Should be excluded for the duration of possible exposure or until they are protected from that disease by immunization

Immunization mandates by state for children in child care and school settings can be found online at www.immunize.org/laws.

Caregiver/Teacher Immunizations

Unless medically contraindicated, immunization is recommended for the following:
- Chickenpox (unless documented to have had the natural disease)
- Hepatitis B virus
- Influenza (annually)
- Measles, mumps, and rubella (unless documented to have had the natural disease)
- Poliomyelitis
- Tetanus and diphtheria (Td), including a Td booster every 10 years

In addition, staff members should be encouraged to receive the following immunizations:
- Pneumococcal polysaccharide (for people 65 years and older)
- Consideration of hepatitis A virus vaccine or, in the event of an outbreak, gamma globulin

If a staff member is not appropriately immunized for medical or religious reasons, the program should require written documentation of the reason.

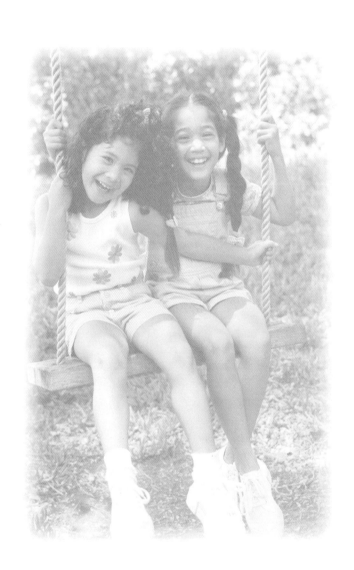

CHAPTER 10

Bioterrorism

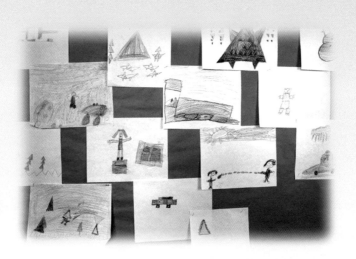

Bioterrorism

It is very unlikely that children in child care and school settings will be the subjects of bioterrorism. However, this information is provided to address any questions that may arise.

Some infectious agents have the potential to be used in acts of bioterrorism. Children may be particularly vulnerable to a bioterrorist attack because, compared with adults, they have a more rapid respiratory rate, increased skin absorption, a higher ratio of skin surface area to weight, and less fluid reserve. Accurate and rapid diagnosis may be more difficult in children because of their inability to describe symptoms. The symptoms of illnesses caused by bioterrorism agents are similar to symptoms of many infectious diseases (eg, fever, malaise, headache, vomiting, diarrhea). Therefore, it will be hard to know when a bioterrorist attack has occurred. If a number of children become ill at the same time, notify your health consultant and the local health department immediately. This will address concerns of bioterrorism as well as the much more likely event of an outbreak of a common community-acquired infectious disease.

Every child care and school setting should have a written disaster plan that should include items specific to bioterrorism.

The following is a list of resources, including Web sites and telephone numbers, that provide updated information concerning clinical recognition, prevention, diagnosis, and treatment of illness caused by potential agents of bioterrorism.

General Information

- State health department Web sites: **www.cdc.gov/other.htm#states**
- Centers for Disease Control and Prevention Emergency Preparedness and Response Web site: **www.bt.cdc.gov**
- American Academy of Pediatrics Children, Terrorism, and Disasters Web site: **www.aap.org/terrorism**

Emergency Contacts

- Centers for Disease Control and Prevention 24-hour notification line: **770/488-7100**
- US Army Medical Research Institute of Infectious Diseases emergency response line: **888/872-7443**
- National Response Center: **800/424-8802** or **202/267-2675**
- Domestic Preparedness help line: **800/368-6498**
- National Disaster Medical System: **800/USA-NDMS (872-6367)** or **ndms.dhhs.gov**

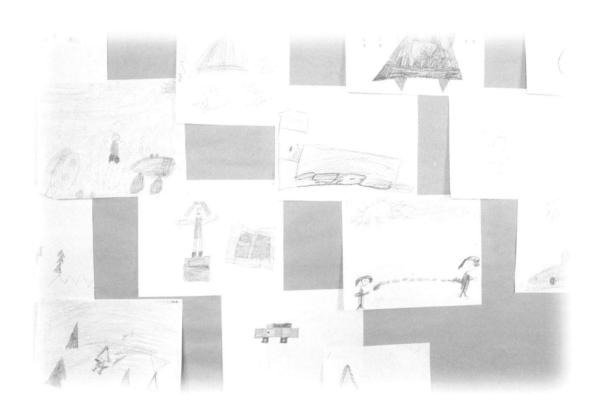

CHAPTER 11

Sample Letters and Forms

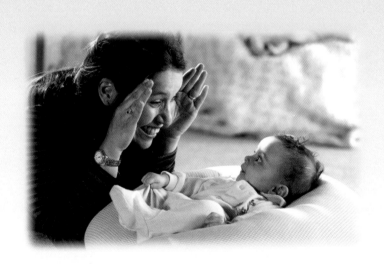

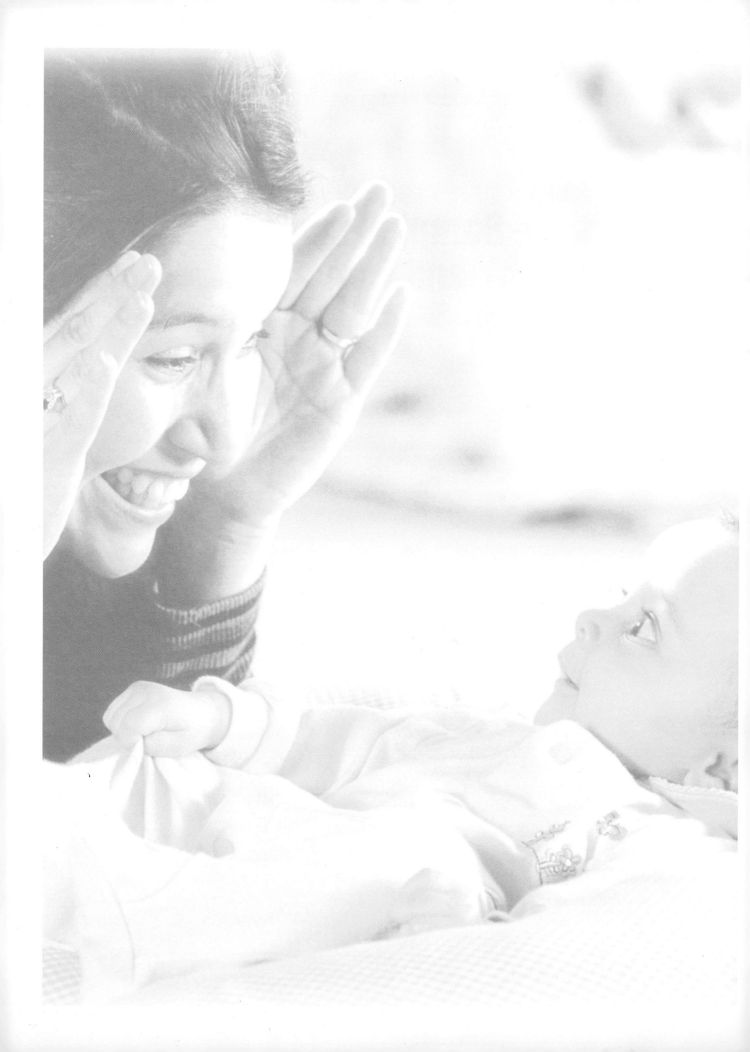

Sample Letters and Forms

Parent/Guardian Alert Letter

Notice of Exposure to Communicable Disease

Name of Facility/School _____

Address of Facility/School _____

Telephone Number of Facility/School _____

Dear Parent or Legal Guardian:

A child in our facility/school has or is suspected of having _____.

We provide you this notice so that you are informed of issues that may affect your child's health in the future. We also want you to understand our facility's/school's exclusion and return-to-care practices for this particular condition. Many communicable diseases do not represent a significant risk to others, nor do they require a health professional visit. Also, in many cases, exclusion of children with certain communicable diseases will not decrease the spread to others. However, for a few, a visit and medical evaluation is essential. Please read the attached information sheet closely and call us with any questions.

_____ at _____
Facility/School Staff Person's Name   Telephone Number

Information About This Disease

Note: To be used if there is no applicable quick reference sheet in Chapter 7. You may copy those pages for communications with families/health professionals.

The disease is spread by _____

The symptoms are _____

_____

_____

_____

The disease can be prevented by _____

_____

_____

What the facility/school is doing to reduce the spread: _____

_____

What you can do at home: _____

_____

_____

_____

Is exclusion necessary? _____

When can an excluded child return? _____

Comments _____

_____

_____

Suspected Illness or Communicable Disease

Name of Child _____

Facility/School _____ Date _____

Dear Parent/Guardian:

Today at our facility/school, your child was observed to have one or more of the following signs or symptoms:

General
- ☐ Fever (101°F or above orally)
- ☐ Headache
- ☐ Swelling of or pus from _____

Eye
- ☐ Pinkeye
- ☐ Tears, redness of eyelid lining

Gastrointestinal
- ☐ Diarrhea (more than one abnormally loose stool)
- ☐ Vomiting

Respiratory
- ☐ Difficult or rapid breathing
- ☐ Severe coughing
- ☐ Child gets red or blue in the face
- ☐ Sore throat or trouble swallowing
- ☐ Earache

Skin
- ☐ Infected skin patches
- ☐ Crusty, bright yellow, dry, or gummy areas of skin
- ☐ Severe itching of body/scalp
- ☐ Unusual spots or rashes
- ☐ Head lice or nits

Unusual behavior
- ☐ Loss of appetite
- ☐ Child cries more than usual
- ☐ Child feels general discomfort
- ☐ Cranky or less active
- ☐ Just seems unwell

Urine problem
- ☐ Specify: _____

Other
- ☐ Specify: _____

Contact your health professional if there is
- ☐ Persistent fever (above 101°F) and child seems very sick
- ☐ Breathing so hard child cannot play, talk, cry, or drink
- ☐ Severe coughing
- ☐ Earache
- ☐ Sore throat with fever
- ☐ Thick nasal drainage that lasts more than 10 days
- ☐ Rash accompanied by fever
- ☐ Persistent diarrhea (more than 1–2 days)
- ☐ Severe headache and stiff neck with fever

- ☐ Yellow skin and/or eyes
- ☐ Considerable confusion or difficult to arouse
- ☐ Rash, hives, or welts that appear quickly
- ☐ Severe stomachache that causes child to double over and scream
- ☐ No urination over 8-hour period; mouth and tongue look dry
- ☐ Black stool or blood mixed with stool
- ☐ Any child who looks or acts very ill or seems to be getting worse quickly

---

We are excluding your child from attendance at our facility/school until (possible options)

☐ The signs or symptoms that required exclusion have resolved.

☐ The child can comfortably participate in normal activities.

☐ We can provide the level of care your child needs.

☐ Other: _____

Parent/Health Professional Release Form

Authorization for Release of Information

I, _____, give permission for
(parent/guardian)

_____
(health professional/facility)

to release to _____ the following information:
(facility/school)

_____.
(screenings, tests, diagnoses, treatments, recommendations)

The information will be used solely to plan and coordinate the care of my child, kept confidential, and only shared with

_____.
(staff title/name)

Name of Child _____

Address _____

City _____ State _____ Zip _____

Date of Birth _____

_____
Parent/Guardian Signature

_____
Witness Signature

_____
Staff Member to Contact for Additional Information

Symptom Record

Name of facility/school _____

Child's name _____

Date _____ Symptom(s) _____

When symptom began, how long it lasted, how severe, how often? _____

_____

Any change in child's behavior? _____

_____

Child's temperature _____ Time taken _____ (Circle one: Armpit   Oral   Rectal   Ear canal)

How much and what type of food and fluid did the child take today? _____

_____

How many urine and bowel movements today and how typical/normal were they? _____

_____

Circle or write in other symptoms.

☐ Runny nose	☐ Sore throat	☐ Cough	☐ Diarrhea
☐ Wheezing	☐ Trouble breathing	☐ Stiff neck	☐ Trouble urinating
☐ Pain	☐ Itching	☐ Trouble sleeping	☐ Earache
☐ Headache	☐ Stomachache	☐ Rash	☐ Vomiting

Other symptoms _____

_____

Any medications today? (name, time, dose) _____

Exposure to chemicals, animals, insects, soaps, or new foods _____

_____

Exposure to other people who were sick (what sickness—for confidentiality reasons, please do not identify individuals)_____

_____

Child's other problems that might affect this illness (eg, asthma, anemia, diabetes, allergy, emotional trauma) _____

_____

What has been done so far? _____

_____

Name of person completing this form _____

Return to Group Care Form

Note: To be used when program staff have questions for a health professional, not for routine return of every excluded or ill child.

Dear Health Care Professional,

_____ *(child's name)* has been excluded from _____ *(name of facility/school)* for the following health reason(s):

Unable to participate in normal activities   _____

Requires more care than the staff can provide   _____

Has a specific acute illness that merits exclusion according to the American Academy of Pediatrics/
American Public Health Association/National Resource Center for Health and Safety in Child Care
(available at nrc.uchsc.edu/CFOC/index.html)   _____

Please assess this child by history and physical examinations (laboratory tests as needed) for
1. The **presence of harmful communicable illness** such as enteric pathogens (eg, *Salmonella, Shigella, Escherichia coli,* campylobacter, *Giardia,* hepatitis A), pertussis, measles, mumps, varicella, rubella, diphtheria, or tuberculosis
2. The **presence of signs or symptoms of severe illness** such as dehydration, respiratory distress, or lethargy
3. The **presence of any condition that would preclude the child from returning** to the routine program or, if a program for ill children is available, what the child needs in the way of care to be able to return while still ill

Please indicate

Harmful communicable disease   No _____   Yes _____

Signs of severe illness   No _____   Yes _____

Condition precluding return   No _____   Yes _____

If yes for any, may return once _____ resolves.

If no for all, may return once
1. Can participate fully in all activities
2. Does not require so much increased supervision that staff cannot properly care for child or other children in the program or school

Please **complete the attached medication administration form** if necessary. Please consider the following suggestions:
• Include acetaminophen or ibuprofen (no medications can be given without orders).
• Avoid "as needed" (prn) orders (these are confusing for caregivers/teachers); instead, describe the signs and symptoms teachers would see that determine when medication should be given.
• Include an asthma action plan for children with asthma.
• Include a care plan for any child with any other chronic condition.

Signature/Stamp _____ Date _____

Thank you for your cooperation.

Request for Medication Administration by Caregivers/Teachers Other Than the Parent

Note: When possible, please reduce or eliminate the need to administer medications in group settings by prescribing medications that can be administered at home.

To: Name of Facility/School _____

Date _____

Child's Name _____

Diagnosis _____

Medication(s) _____

_____

Dosage(s) _____

_____

Time(s) of Administration _____

_____

Special Instructions for Method to Use in Administering Medication(s) and
Who the Facility/School Can Call for Training in Any Special Techniques _____

_____

_____

Possible Side Effects _____

_____

_____

I hereby give permission for the facility/school to administer medication as prescribed above. I also give permission for the caregiver/teacher to contact the prescribing pediatric health professional about the administration of this medication.

_____
Parent or Guardian Signature

_____
Home Phone   Work Phone   Cell Phone

_____
Prescribing Health Professional's Name   Prescribing Health Professional's Phone Number

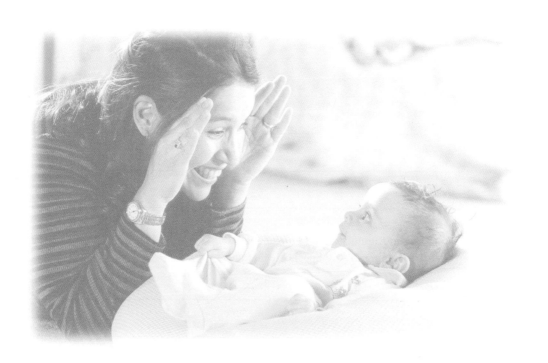

Glossary

These definitions are adapted from American Academy of Pediatrics, American Public Health Association, National Resource Center for Health and Safety in Child Care. *Caring for Our Children: National Health and Safety Performance Standards: Guidelines for Out-of-Home Child Care Programs.* 2nd ed. Elk Grove Village, IL: American Academy of Pediatrics; 2002. Available at: http://nrc.uchsc.edu/CFOC/index.html. Accessed August 13, 2004.

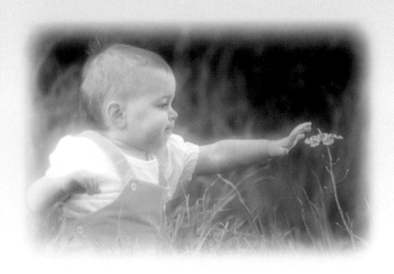

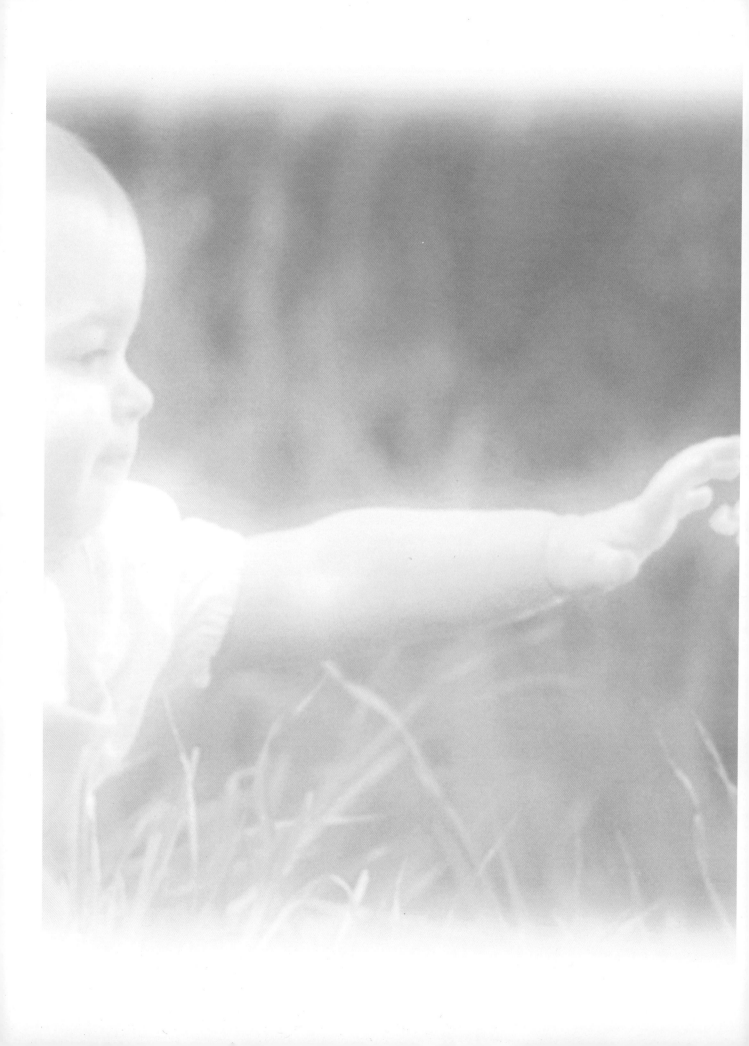

Glossary

AAP: Abbreviation for the American Academy of Pediatrics, a national organization of pediatricians founded in 1930 and dedicated to the improvement of child health and welfare.

Acute: Adjective describing an illness that has a sudden onset and is of short duration.

Adult-child ratio: The maximum number of children permitted per caregiver/teacher.

Antibiotic prophylaxis: Antibiotics that are prescribed to prevent infections in infants and children in situations associated with an increased risk of serious infection with a specific disease.

APHA: Abbreviation for the American Public Health Association, a national organization of health professionals that protects and promotes the health of the public through education, research, advocacy, and policy development.

Assessment: An in-depth appraisal conducted to diagnose a condition or determine the importance or value of a procedure.

Bacteria: Plural of bacterium. Organisms that may be responsible for localized or generalized diseases and can survive in and out of the body. They are much larger than viruses and usually can be treated effectively with antibiotics.

Bleach solution: For sanitizing environmental surfaces—use a spray solution of one-quarter (¼) cup of household liquid chlorine bleach (sodium hypochlorite) in 1 gallon of water, prepared fresh daily. See also *Disinfect.*

Body fluids: Urine, feces, saliva, blood, nasal discharge, eye discharge, and injury or tissue discharge.

Bronchitis: Most often a bacterial or viral infection that causes swelling of the tubes (bronchi) leading to the lungs.

Caregiver: Used here to indicate the primary staff who work directly with the children, ie, director, teacher, aide, or others in the center and child care provider in small and large family child care homes and in schools.

Carrier: A person who carries within his or her body a specific disease-causing organism, has no symptoms of disease, and can spread the disease to others. For example, some children may be carriers of *Haemophilus influenzae* or *Giardia* and have no symptoms.

CDC: Abbreviation for the Centers for Disease Control and Prevention, which is responsible for monitoring communicable diseases, immunization status, injuries, and congenital malformations and performing other disease and injury surveillance activities in the United States.

Center: A facility that provides care and education for any number of children in a nonresidential setting and is open on a regular basis (ie, it is not a drop-in facility).

Children with special needs: Children who have or are at increased risk for a chronic physical, developmental, behavioral, or emotional condition and who also require health and related services of a type or amount beyond that required by children generally.

Chronic: Adjective describing an infection or illness that lasts a long time (months or years).

Clean: To remove dirt and debris (eg, blood, urine, feces) by scrubbing and washing with a detergent solution and rinsing with water.

Communicable disease: A disease caused by a microorganism (eg, bacterium, virus, fungus, parasite) that can be transmitted from person to person via an infected body fluid or respiratory spray, with or without an intermediary agent (eg, louse, mosquito) or environmental object (eg, table surface). Many communicable diseases are reportable to the local health authority.

Compliance: The act of carrying out a recommendation, policy, or procedure.

Contamination: The presence of infectious microorganisms in or on the body, environmental surfaces, articles of clothing, or food or water.

Contraindication: Something (eg, symptom, condition) that makes a particular treatment or procedure inadvisable.

Croup: Spasms of the airway that cause difficult breathing and a cough sounding like a seal's bark. Croup can be caused by various bacteria and viruses.

Dermatitis: An inflammation of the skin caused by irritation or infection.

Diphtheria: A serious infection of the nose and throat caused by the bacterium *Corynebacterium diphtheriae,* producing symptoms of sore throat, low fever, chills, and a grayish membrane in the throat. The membrane can make swallowing and breathing difficult and may cause suffocation. The bacteria produce a toxin (a type of poisonous substance) that can cause severe and permanent damage to the nervous system and heart. This infection has been almost entirely eliminated in areas where standard infant immunizations and boosters are performed.

Disinfect: To eliminate virtually all germs from inanimate surfaces through the use of chemicals (eg, products registered with the US Environmental Protection Agency as "disinfectants") or physical agents (eg, heat).

Enteric: Describes the location of infections affecting the intestines (often with diarrhea) or liver.

EPA: Abbreviation for the US Environmental Protection Agency, established in 1970, which administers federal programs on air and water pollution, solid waste disposal, pesticide regulation, and radiation and noise control.

Epiglottis: Tissue lid of the voice box. When this organ becomes swollen and inflamed (a condition called epiglottitis), it can block breathing passages. *Haemophilus influenzae* type b commonly causes epiglottitis. This infection has been greatly reduced in areas where standard infant immunizations and boosters are performed.

Evaluation: Impressions and recommendations formed after a careful appraisal and study.

Exclusion: Denying admission of an ill child or staff member to a facility.

Excretion: Waste material that is formed and not used by the body (eg, feces, urine).

Facility: A legal definition of the buildings, grounds, equipment, and people involved in providing child care of any type.

Febrile: The condition of having an abnormally high body temperature (fever), often as a response to infection.

Fever: An elevation of body temperature. Body temperature can be elevated by overheating caused by overdressing or a hot environment, reactions to medications, and response to infection. For this purpose, fever is defined as temperature above 101°F orally, above 102°F rectally, or 100°F or higher taken axillary (armpit) or measured by any equivalent method. Fever is an indication of the body's response to something, but is neither a disease nor a serious problem by itself.

Fungi: Plural of fungus. Plantlike organisms such as yeasts, molds, mildew, and mushrooms that get their nutrition from other living organisms or dead organic matter.

Germ: A small mass of living substance capable of developing into an organism or one of its parts.

Group A streptococcus: Bacterium commonly found in the throat and on the skin that can cause a range of infections, from relatively mild sore throats and skin infections to life-threatening diseases.

Group care setting: A facility where children from more than one family receive care together.

HBV: Abbreviation for hepatitis B virus.

Health care professional: Practices medicine by an established licensing body with or without supervision. The most common types of health care professionals include physicians, nurse practitioners, and physician assistants.

Health consultant: A physician, certified pediatric or family nurse practitioner, registered nurse, or environmental, oral, mental health, nutrition, or other health professional who has pediatric and child care experience and is knowledgeable in pediatric health practice, child care, licensing, and community resources. The health consultant provides guidance and assistance to child care staff on health aspects of the facility.

Hib: Abbreviation for *Haemophilus influenzae* type b.

HIV: Abbreviation for human immunodeficiency virus.

Hygiene: Protective measures taken by individuals to promote health and limit the spread of infectious diseases.

Immune globulin (gamma globulin, immunoglobulin): An antibody preparation made from human plasma. Provides temporary protection against diseases such as hepatitis A. Health officials may wish to give doses of immune globulin to children in child care when cases of hepatitis appear.

Immunity: The body's ability to fight a particular infection. For example, a child acquires immunity to diseases such as measles, mumps, rubella, and pertussis after natural infection or by immunization. Newborn children initially have the same immune status as their mothers. This immunity usually disappears within the first 6 months of life.

Immunizations: Vaccines that are given to children and adults to help them develop protection (antibodies) against specific infections. Vaccines may contain an inactivated or killed agent or a weakened live organism.

Impervious: Not allowing entrance or passage; impenetrable.

Incubation period: Time between exposure to an infectious microorganism and beginning of symptoms.

Infant: A child between the time of birth and age of ambulation (usually between birth and 18 months).

Infection: A condition caused by the multiplication of an infectious agent in the body.

Infectious: Capable of causing an infection.

Infestation: Common usage of this term refers to parasites (eg, lice, scabies) living on the outside of the body.

Ingestion: The act of taking material (whether food or other substances) into the body through the mouth.

Intradermal: Relating to areas between the layers of the skin (as in intradermal injections).

Jaundice: Yellowish discoloration of the whites of the eyes, skin, and mucous membranes caused by deposition of bile salts in these tissues. It occurs as a symptom of various diseases such as hepatitis that affect the processing of bile.

Lethargy: Unusual sleepiness.

Mantoux intradermal skin test: Involves the intradermal injection of a standardized amount of tuberculin antigen. The reaction to the antigen on the skin can be measured and the result used to assess the likelihood of infection with tuberculosis.

Medications: Any substances that are intended to diagnose, cure, treat, or prevent disease or affect the structure or function of the body of humans or other animals.

MMR: Abbreviation for the vaccine against measles, mumps, and rubella.

Organisms: Living things. Often used as a general term for germs (eg, bacteria, viruses, fungi, parasites) that can cause disease.

OSHA: Abbreviation for the Occupational Safety and Health Administration of the US Department of Labor, which regulates health and safety in the workplace.

Parasite: An organism that lives on or in another living organism (eg, tick, louse, mite).

Parent: The child's natural or adoptive mother or father, guardian, or other legally responsible person.

Pesticides: Chemicals used to kill pests, particularly insects.

Poliomyelitis: A disease caused by the polio virus with signs that may include paralysis and meningitis but often only include minor flu-like symptoms. This infection has been almost entirely eliminated in areas where standard infant immunizations and boosters are performed.

RSV: Abbreviation for respiratory syncytial virus.

Rhinovirus: A virus that causes the common cold.

Sanitize: To remove filth or soil and small amounts of certain bacteria. For an inanimate surface to be considered sanitary, the surface must be clean (see *Clean*) and the number of germs must be reduced to such a level that disease transmission by that surface is unlikely. This procedure is less rigorous than disinfection (see *Disinfect*) and is applicable to a wide variety of routine housekeeping procedures involving, for example, bedding, bathrooms, kitchen countertops, floors, and walls.

Screening: Mass examination of a population group to detect the existence of a particular disease (eg, diabetes, tuberculosis).

Secretions: Wet materials such as saliva that are produced by cells or glands and have a specific purpose in the body.

Seizure: A sudden attack or convulsion caused by involuntary, uncontrolled bursts of electrical activity in the brain that can result in a wide variety of clinical manifestations including muscle twitches, staring, tongue biting, loss of consciousness, and total body shaking.

Staff: Used here to indicate all personnel employed at the child care facility or school, including caregivers, teachers, and personnel who do not provide direct care to children (eg, cooks, drivers, housekeeping personnel).

Standard precautions: Apply to contact with non-intact skin, mucous membranes, blood, all body fluids, and excretions except sweat, whether they contain visible blood. The general methods of infection prevention are indicated for all people in the group care setting and designed to reduce the risk of transmission of microorganisms from recognized and unrecognized sources of infection. Although standard precautions were designed to apply to hospital settings, with the exceptions detailed in this definition, they also apply in group care settings. Standard precautions involve use of barriers against spread of blood-borne disease as in universal precautions (see *Universal precautions*) as well as cleaning and sanitizing surfaces contaminated by other body fluids.

Group care adaptation of standard precautions (exceptions from the use in hospital settings) are as follows:

- Use of nonporous gloves is optional except when blood or blood-containing body fluids may be involved.
- Gowns and masks are not required.
- Appropriate barriers include materials such as disposable diaper table paper and disposable towels and surfaces that can be sanitized in group care settings.

Streptococcus: A common bacterium that can cause sore throat, upper respiratory illnesses, pneumonia, skin rashes, skin infections, arthritis, heart disease (rheumatic fever), and kidney disease (glomerulonephritis).

Substitute staff: Caregivers/teachers (often without prior training or experience) hired for one day or an extended period.

TB: Abbreviation for tuberculosis.

Toddler: A child between the age of ambulation and toilet learning/training (usually between 13 and 35 months).

Transmission: The passing of an infectious organism or germ from person to person.

Under-immunized: A person who has not received the recommended number or types of vaccines for his or her age according to the current national and local immunization schedules.

Universal precautions: Apply to blood and other body fluids containing blood, semen, and vaginal secretions, but not to feces, nasal secretions, sputum, sweat, tears, urine, saliva, and vomitus, unless they contain visible blood or are likely to contain blood. Universal precautions include avoiding injuries caused by sharp instruments or devices and the use of protective barriers such as gloves, gowns, aprons, masks, or protective eyewear, which can reduce the risk of exposure of the worker's skin or mucous membranes that could come in contact with materials that may contain blood-borne pathogens while the worker is providing first aid or care.

Virus: A microscopic organism, smaller than a bacterium, that may cause disease. Viruses can grow or reproduce only in living cells.

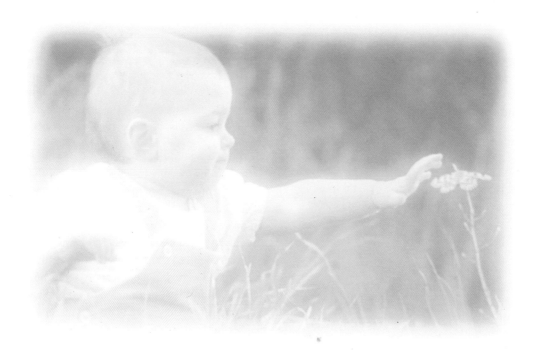